The NHS in England 2004/05: a pocket guide

Peter Davies

£12.95

First, second, third, fourth, fifth and sixth editions published by:

The NHS Confederation
1 Warwick Row,
London SW1E 5ER
Tel 020 7959 7272
Fax 020 7959 7273

To order further copies of this Guide or other Confederation publications, contact our publications sales team on 0870 444 5841 or visit www.nhsconfed.org/publications

ISBN 1 85947 101 3
Printed in the UK.

The sixth edition of The *NHS in England 2004/05: a pocket guide.*

BOK 54901

Contents

Foreword 1

1 First principles 3

2 The structure of the NHS 5

Parliament 6

The Department of Health 6

Special health authorities 14

Strategic health authorities 14

Primary care trusts 16

NHS trusts 17

Foundation trusts 18

Care trusts 19

Children's trusts 19

Managed clinical networks 20

The role of boards 23

3 Where care is delivered 28

Primary care 28

Intermediate care 33

Secondary care 34

Mental health 38

Involving patients and the public 41

4 NHS strategy: putting policy in context 47

The planning framework 49

Priorities 2003–06 53

5 NHS quality: improving healthcare 54

Organisations' responsibility for quality 54

Healthcare professions' responsibility for quality 66

Feedback from patients 72
Complaints 73

6 Financing the NHS 76
Sources of funding 76
Resource allocation 79
Capital 83
NHS spending 86

7 Human resources 93
Staff numbers 93
The importance of good HR in health services 96
Training 98
NHSU 99
Pay 103
Workforce planning 109

8 Information technology in the NHS 113
National Programme for IT 114
The electronic NHS 118

9 Public sector partnerships 121
Local authorities 123
Other partnerships 126
Public health 128

10 Research and development 137
DoH policy research programme 137
NHS R&D programme 138

11 The NHS: a brief history 141

12 An A–Z of the NHS 147

13 Acronym buster 157

Index 164

Foreword

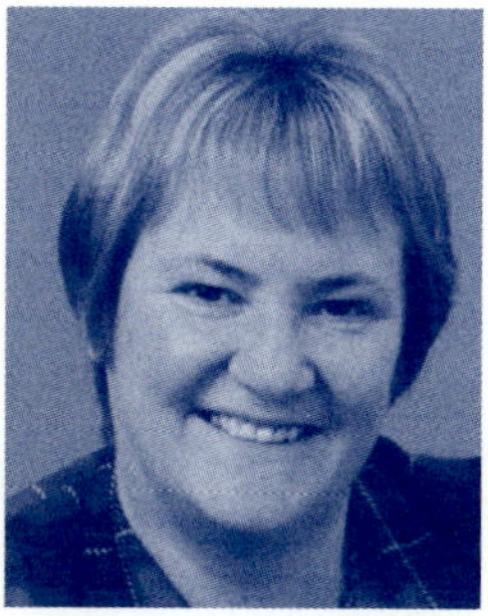

Welcome to the 2004/05 edition of the NHS Confederation's *Pocket guide to the NHS in England*.

Many of the Government's radical plans for the NHS are now becoming reality. There are, however, still many more changes on the horizon. To help you understand these changes and their relevance to your organisation we have completely revised and updated the guide for this year. *The NHS in England 2004/05: a pocket guide* provides an insight into the latest health service developments as well as a truly comprehensive introduction to the NHS.

I am delighted that Peter Davies, former editor of the *Health Service Journal*, has written this new edition for us. Peter is a widely-published writer and contributes a regular column on health policy to the *Guardian* website. He has been able to make use of the expertise of the Confederation's policy team to make this edition of the *Pocket guide* essential reading for anyone involved with the health service.

Whether you are an NHS veteran, new to this vast and complex organisation, or working in partnership with it, I think the *Pocket guide* will prove an indispensable reference tool. If you have any comments or suggestions for areas you would like covered in future editions, please contact our publications department on 020 7959 7266 or at publications@nhsconfed.org

I would like to thank NHSU for kindly supporting this edition of the *Pocket guide*.

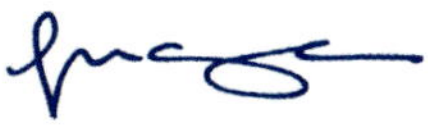

Dr Gill Morgan
Chief Executive
The NHS Confederation

The NHS Confederation

The NHS Confederation brings together the organisations that make up the NHS across the UK. Working with our members, we are an independent driving force to transform health services and health by:

- influencing policy and the wider public debate
- connecting health leaders through networking and information sharing.

How do we influence?

The Confederation works in three interrelated ways:

- through leading-edge thinking, drawing on the cutting-edge ideas and practice of our members, and acting as a catalyst to generate new thinking
- informing current policy by feeding the perspective of members into the development of policy and its implementation
- shaping the wider climate of opinion by engaging the media, politicians and other opinion-formers in robust dialogue, while ensuring that the realities and achievements of the NHS are reflected in the public debate.

How do we connect?

The Confederation supports networking and the sharing of information within and beyond the NHS through:

- events, meetings and forums, from our annual conference and exhibition to national conferences, and from regional events to policy development seminars
- publishing, from reports on Government policy developments and briefings specifically tailored for non-executives to our popular pocket guides to the NHS
- initiatives, such as the Future Healthcare Network for NHS organisations actively involved in PFI and LIFT, the Nexus programme for non-executives, and the associate subscription service, for organisations working alongside the NHS.

1 First principles

The principles on which the NHS rests originate in the 1940s, when it was founded. The 1944 white paper, *A National health service*, stated that:

> The government want to ensure that in future every man, woman and child can rely on getting all the advice and treatment and care they may need in matters of personal health; that what they shall get shall be the best medical and other facilities available; that their getting these shall not depend on whether they can pay for them or any other factor irrelevant to the real need.

Both society and the health service have altered almost beyond recognition since then, but the NHS still strives to provide a broadly comprehensive service, mostly free to all at the point of need. Of course, it has had to move with the times to take advantage of scientific and technological advances, as well as political, social and economic change. The current Government set out the basis for its extensive reform programme in the NHS Plan, published in 2000. That document contained ten core principles to underpin the service and the reforms, agreed after discussion with NHS staff, patients and others. Some echo the NHS's founding principles, others reflect today's important issues.

NHS core principles

- The NHS will provide a universal service for all, based on clinical need, not ability to pay.
- The NHS will provide a comprehensive range of services.
- The NHS will shape its services around the needs and preferences of individual patients, their families and their carers.
- The NHS will respond to different needs of different populations.
- The NHS will work continuously to improve quality services and to minimise errors.
- The NHS will support and value its staff.
- Public funds for healthcare will be devoted solely to NHS patients.
- The NHS will work together with others to ensure a seamless service for patients.
- The NHS will help keep people healthy and work to reduce health inequalities.

- The NHS will respect the confidentiality of individual patients and provide open access to information about services, treatment and performance.

Since the Plan was published, the Government has continued to develop NHS policy. It wants the service to offer patients a choice of where and when they are treated, and is keen to devolve decision making from Whitehall to local level, with primary care in particular taking a leading role. Perhaps most radically, it is encouraging 'plurality of provision' in healthcare, with the private and voluntary sectors treating NHS patients on a much larger scale than they have done before. This begins to redefine what is meant by a national health service: it will be not a monopoly provider of care but a system of diverse providers united by common principles – in particular, providing comprehensive services to all, free at the point of need.

Health Secretary John Reid has described the philosophy and values that will guide his implementation of the reforms, emphasising four fundamental principles:

- Healthcare should be provided equally to those who need it, free at the point of need.
- The NHS is defined around the needs of the patients.
- The NHS must increase its comprehensive capacity as well as increase the choice and diversity it offers patients.
- Equity – fairness – is the cornerstone of the NHS, particularly equality of access.

Elaborating on these principles in his first major speech as Health Secretary – to the NHS Confederation's annual conference in 2003 – Dr Reid said that introducing new healthcare providers was essential for strengthening capacity and choice. He added: 'The aim of the 1948 health service to provide equality of access to healthcare has not been fully met.' Recognising and rectifying this was vital to creating the 'personalised health service' that is the ultimate aim of the NHS reforms.

2 The structure of the NHS

Parliament

As the NHS is financed mainly through taxation it relies on Parliament for its funds, and has to account to Parliament for their use through the Secretary of State for Health, the cabinet member responsible for the service. Parliament scrutinises the service through debates, MPs' questions to ministers and select committees. These procedures mean that the Government has to publicly explain and defend its policies for the NHS.

Select committees

Three select committees, each comprising backbench MPs representing the major parties, are particularly relevant to the NHS. They are all able to summon ministers, civil servants and NHS employees to give oral or written evidence to their inquiries, usually in public. Their reports are published throughout the parliamentary session.

Health committee

The health committee's role is 'to examine the expenditure, administration and policy of the Department of Health and its associated bodies'. It has a maximum of 11 members. Recent inquiries have covered choice and inequalities in maternity services, patient and public involvement in the NHS and foundation trusts.
www.parliament.uk/parliamentary_committees/health_committee.cfm

Public accounts committee

The public accounts committee is concerned with ensuring the NHS is operating with economy, efficiency and effectiveness. Its inquiries are based on reports about the service's 'value for money', produced by the Comptroller and Auditor General, who heads the National Audit Office. It aims to draw lessons from past successes and failures that can be applied to future activity. The committee has 16 members, and is traditionally chaired by a member of the Opposition.
www.parliament.uk/parliamentary_committees/committee_of_public_accounts.cfm
www.nao.gov.uk

Public administration committee

The public administration committee examines reports from the Health Service Commissioner (better known as the Ombudsman, see page 75). It has 11 members.
www.parliament.uk/parliamentary_committees/public_administration_select_committee.cfm
www.ombudsman.org.uk

Health ministers

The Department of Health has six ministers: the Secretary of State, two ministers of state and three parliamentary under-secretaries of state, one of whom is responsible for public health matters and one for social and community services, while the third sits in the House of Lords. The Secretary of State has overall strategic responsibility for NHS improvement, delivery, reform, finance and resources, while the other ministers each have specific areas of NHS activity assigned to them. The Department for Education and Skills has the lead for children's issues and works closely with the Department of Health.

The Department of Health

The role of the Department of Health (DoH) is to support the Government in improving the health and well-being of the population. It is responsible for the NHS, social services and public health. It negotiates levels of NHS funding with the Treasury, and allocates resources to the health service at large. Setting national standards for the health service has become an important part of its remit.
The organisation is divided into three business groups:

- standards and quality
- strategy and business development
- delivery.

The DoH is based in London and Leeds.
www.dh.gov.uk

The structure of the Department of Health

Health & Social Care Standards & Quality

- Health Protection, International Health & Scientific Development
- Research & Development
- Health Improvement
- Quality & Standards
- Care Services
- Regional Public Health
- Group Business Team

Strategy & Business Development

Corporate Management & Development

- Corporate Human Resources
- Information Services
- Customer Services
- Medicines, Pharmacy & Industry
- Secretariat

Communications

- Media Centre
- Campaign Management
- Strategy Policy & Communications
- Programmes & Planning

User Experience & Involvement

- Improving Patient Experience Programme
- The Professions

Strategy

- Statement Unit
- Corporate Analytical Centre
- Customer Intelligence
- Systems & Policy Development

Health & Social Care Services Delivery

- Access
- Finance & Investment
- Workforce
- International Systems & National Programme Delivery
- Programmes & Performance
- Group Business Team

The DoH board

The departmental board manages the DoH's business and priorities. Board members are:

- permanent secretary and NHS chief executive
- group director, delivery
- group director, standards and quality, and chief medical officer
- group director, strategy and business development
- director of finance and investment
- director of communications
- director of user experience and involvement, and chief nursing officer.

The permanent secretary and NHS chief executive

These two roles, formerly separate, were combined in 2000. The holder is directly responsible to the Secretary of State for the service's management and performance. The chief executive's report to the NHS is published in December each year and outlines the service's progress towards meeting key objectives. The chief executive produces a weekly bulletin, e-mailed every Thursday to NHS and council chief executives and directors of social services, containing details of publications, circulars and announcements.
www.publications.doh.gov.uk/nhsreport/index.htm
www.publications.doh.gov.uk/cebulletin/index.htm

The chief medical officer and heads of profession

Seven heads of profession currently provide expert knowledge on health and social care:

- chief medical officer
- chief nursing officer
- chief dental officer
- chief social services inspector
- chief health professions officer
- chief pharmaceutical officer
- chief scientist.

The chief medical officer (CMO) is the Government's principal medical adviser and the professional head of all medical staff in England. The CMO produces an annual independent report on the state of the nation's health.

National clinical directors

National clinical directors are experts in their field and take the lead in implementing key national clinical priorities. Their roles vary but include chairing taskforces, promoting the work of their specialism, developing clinical networks and advising on clinical quality and governance. They are:

- national director for emergency access
- national director for mental health
- national clinical director for children
- national director for heart disease
- national clinical director for primary care
- national director for older people's services
- national cancer director
- national clinical director for diabetes.

The Modernisation Board

The Modernisation Board's role is to ensure 'real and speedy progress' in implementing the NHS Plan. It aims to smooth obstacles to change and encourage the right people to work together. Members include representatives of professional bodies, medical Royal Colleges and patient groups as well as practising clinicians and NHS managers. It is chaired by the health secretary and also includes the NHS chief executive.

The NHS Modernisation Agency

The agency's role has been to support the NHS and its partner organisations in modernising services to meet the needs and convenience of patients. Set up in April 2001, its focus has been mainly on improving access, increasing local support, raising standards, and sharing knowledge widely. The agency has sought to make modernisation mainstream, working closely with strategic health authorities.

The agency's future role and size is being discussed as part of the DoH's change programme (see page 12), and its new structure will be finalised after a review. If it is decided to reduce the agency's 760 staff, most modernisation work would then be done at local level. www.modern.nhs.uk

The agency's main components are:

NHS Leadership Centre – charged with developing current and future leaders and managers at all levels and from across the professions.

New Ways of Working Team – aims to ensure the NHS has sufficient numbers of trained, motivated staff through better skills utilisation (see page 111).

NHS Clinical Governance Support Team – helps organisations implement clinical governance (see page 55) with information, advice and development programmes. It works with challenged organisations to develop and maintain improvements to their services. It is also involved in promoting public and patient involvement and improving the patient experience.
www.cgsupport.nhs.uk

Innovation and Knowledge Group – helps organisations explore and develop tools, techniques and innovative approaches to change.

Technology in Health Group – helps strategic health authorities realise the benefits of the national IT programme.

National Institute for Mental Health in England – provides local development centres and national programmes with help to implement policy and resolve local challenges in developing mental health services. Launched in 2002, NIMHE takes a lead in connecting mental health research, development, delivery, monitoring and review.
www.nimhe.org.uk

National Primary Care Development Team – is affiliated to the Modernisation Agency, and specialises in helping individuals and organisations achieve rapid, systematic and sustainable improvements in primary care. Its 11 centres engage patients and frontline clinicians in improvement work.
www.npdt.org

National and Primary Care Trust Development Programme – provides organisational development support to every primary care trust and strategic health authority. NatPaCT works with challenged PCTs and health economies through the PCT improvement programme.
www.natpact.nhs.uk

Service Improvement Team – focuses on improving access to hospital services by reducing waiting times and introducing booked appointments.

Partnership Development Group – aims to ensure the agency is well integrated with its partner organisations. Set up in 2003, it is concentrating on relationships with strategic health authorities initially, but will focus on how the agency links to the DoH, the National Institute for Clinical Excellence (NICE) and the Healthcare Commission (formerly CHAI).

Executive agencies

Five executive agencies within the DoH are responsible for particular business areas. They are:

Health Protection Agency – is dedicated to protecting people's health and reducing the impact of infectious diseases, chemical hazards, poisons and radiation hazards (see page 131).

Medicines and Healthcare Products Regulatory Agency – protects public health and patient safety by ensuring that medicines, healthcare products and medical equipment meet safety and effectiveness standards, and are used safely.
www.mhra.gov.uk

NHS Estates – provides advice on healthcare buildings and facilities (see page 37).

NHS Pensions Agency – is the administration centre for the NHS pension scheme, which has 1.6 million members.
www.nhspa.gov.uk

NHS Purchasing and Supply Agency – advises on procurement policy and strategy, and contracts nationally for products and services critical to the NHS, using its purchasing power to achieve savings (see page 92).

Non-departmental government bodies

These exist across government, and are set up when ministers want independent advice without direct influence from Whitehall departments. They fall into three categories:

Commissions have a role in national government but are not formally part of any department. They include the Healthcare Commission, General Social Care Council, Human Fertilisation and Embryology Authority and National Radiological Protection Board.

Advisory bodies number more than 30 and include the Expert Advisory Group on AIDS, the Nutrition Forum and the Joint Committee on Vaccination and Immunisation.

Tribunals are created by legislation and make decisions in specialised fields of law. They are the Care Standards Tribunal, Family Health Services Appeal Authority, Mental Health Review Tribunals and the Registered Homes Tribunal.

Reform and the DoH

The DoH is engaged in an 18-month change programme that will reduce its core staff by almost 40 per cent to 2,200 by October 2004. About half the posts will be abolished, and half transferred to arm's-length bodies. This reflects the Government's drive to shift power from Whitehall to frontline healthcare staff. The DoH's new role will be to provide strategic leadership to NHS and social care organisations, concentrating on:

- setting overall direction
- ensuring national standards are set
- securing resources
- making major investment decisions
- driving choice for patients and users.

A review of the DoH's arm's-length bodies, many of which are mentioned on the previous page – which employ over 19,000 people – is to look in detail at their role, how efficiently they operate and how they can reduce demands on frontline services.

In addition, as part of the Lyons review of public sector relocation, the DoH has proposed moving about 1,000 posts from its arm's-length bodies away from London and the South East by 2008, with about 600 of them relocating to Leeds. A further 80 core DoH posts would also be relocated. If all the proposals are implemented, 32 per cent of staff in the DoH and its arm's-length bodies would remain in London and the South East.

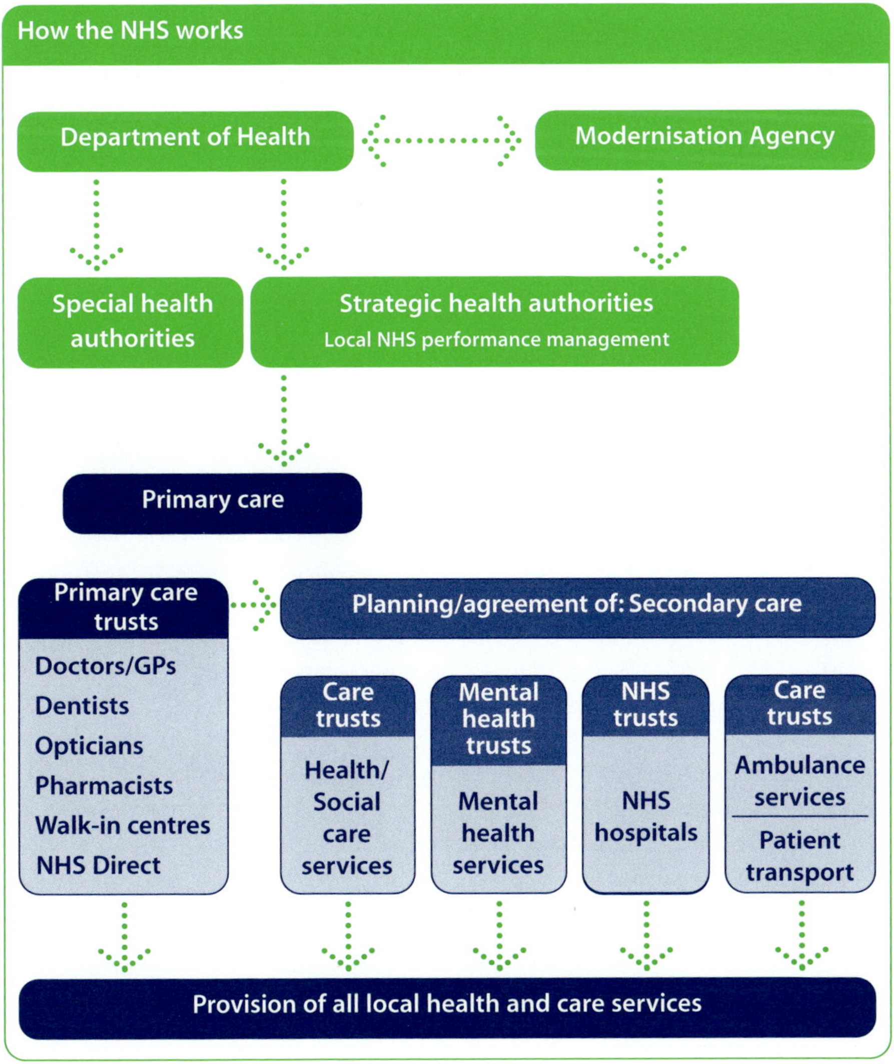
How the NHS works
Department of Health
Modernisation Agency
Special health authorities
Strategic health authorities
Local NHS performance management
Primary care
Primary care trusts
Doctors/GPs
Dentists
Opticians
Pharmacists
Walk-in centres
NHS Direct
Planning/agreement of: Secondary care
Care trusts
Health/ Social care services
Mental health trusts
Mental health services
NHS trusts
NHS hospitals
Care trusts
Ambulance services
Patient transport
Provision of all local health and care services

Special health authorities

Special health authorities provide a service to the whole of England rather than to a local community. They are independent, but can be subject to ministerial direction like other NHS bodies. They currently number 19 and include, for example:

- Mental Health Act Commission
- National Blood Authority
- Prescription Pricing Authority
- UK Transplant.

Strategic health authorities

The 28 strategic health authorities (SHAs) manage the NHS locally on behalf of the DoH, each covering an average population of 1.8 million. Their three key functions are:

- creating a coherent strategic framework
- agreeing annual performance agreements, and performance management of primary care trusts and NHS trusts
- building capacity and supporting performance improvement.

They develop strategies for capital investment, information management and workforce development. Where problems or conflicts arise between local NHS organisations, SHAs will broker solutions. They foster partnerships with non-NHS bodies, universities and further education institutions, as well as help local authorities' overview and scrutiny committees monitor the health service. SHAs must ensure consultation on major service reconfigurations.

Strategic health authority areas

1 Avon, Gloucestershire and Wiltshire
2 Bedfordshire and Hertfordshire
3 Birmingham and the Black Country
4 Cheshire and Merseyside
5 County Durham and Tees Valley
6 Coventry, Warwickshire, Herefordshire and Worcestershire
7 Cumbria and Lancashire
8 Essex
9 Greater Manchester
10 Hampshire and Isle of Wight
11 Kent and Medway
12 Leicestershire, Northamptonshire and Rutland

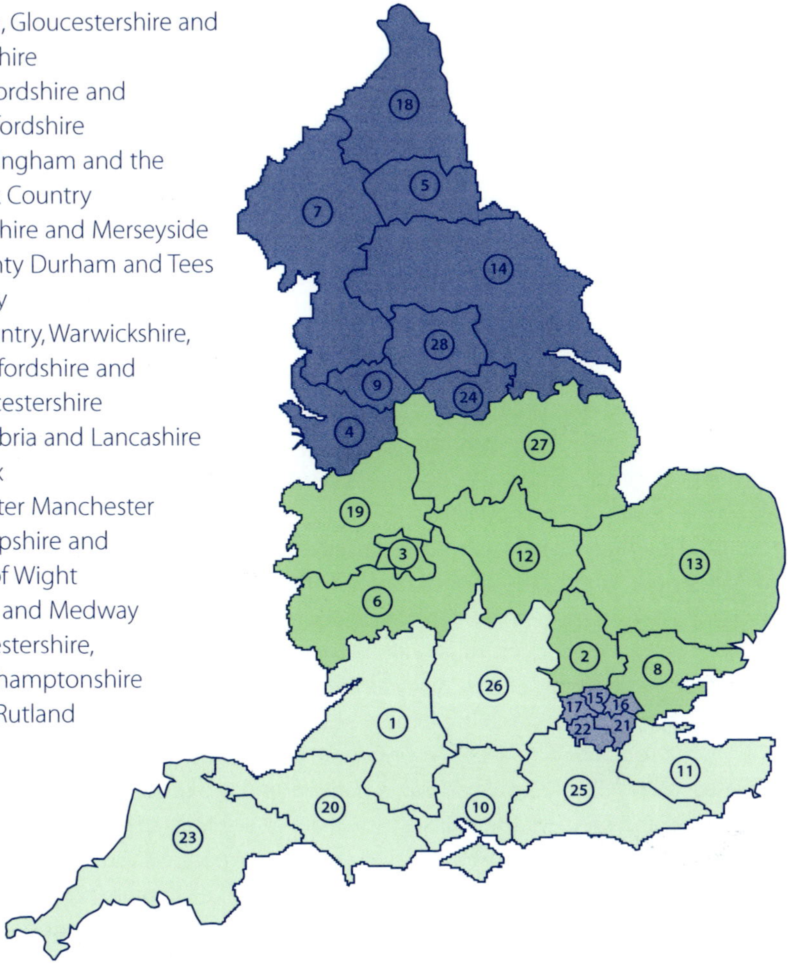

13 Norfolk, Suffolk and Cambridgeshire
14 North and East Yorkshire and Northern Lincolnshire
15 North Central London
16 North East London
17 North West London
18 Northumberland, Tyne and Wear
19 Shropshire and Staffordshire
20 Somerset and Dorset
21 South East London
22 South West London
23 South West Peninsula
24 South Yorkshire
25 Surrey and Sussex
26 Thames Valley
27 Trent
28 West Yorkshire

Primary care trusts

Primary care trusts (PCTs) are the cornerstone of the NHS locally: they run primary and community services and commission secondary care. There are 303 PCTs, serving populations of 170,000 on average. It is the Government's wish that the health service should be 'primary care-led', arguing that primary care staff are uniquely placed to have an overview of hospital and community services, of public health and health services and of local authorities and the NHS. Reflecting this, from 2004 PCTs control 75 per cent of the NHS budget.

PCTs have three main functions:

- improving the health of the community – assessing its health needs and preparing plans, tackling health inequalities, leading partnership working with local authorities and others
- developing primary and community health services – managing and integrating all medical, dental, pharmaceutical and optical primary and community services, as well as ensuring their quality
- commissioning hospital care – either singly or in partnership with other organisations where they cannot be self-sufficient (see below).

They are responsible for commissioning all acute and specialised care, as well as services for mental health, emergency ambulances and patient transport, NHS Direct and walk-in centres. They also implement population screening programmes.

PCTs must work collaboratively, involving patients and the public as well as their own GP practices and partners. They must co-ordinate all agencies delivering healthcare in their area, taking responsibility for creating strong local partnerships to address the broader influences on health, and be ready to work with each other across boundaries. Strategic health authorities are responsible for managing PCTs' performance.

Commissioning

PCTs make most commissioning decisions. They must first identify their population's health needs, then work with potential healthcare providers to develop a service to meet those needs. The results can range from large contracts for acute care in hospitals to small contracts with voluntary sector providers.

Joint commissioning brings together PCTs and social care services for strategic planning and development of services, using their resources collaboratively for the best outcomes.

Commissioning specialised services – usually in low volume, but with high costs – such as those for rare cancers, which only a small number of centres provide, is done by PCTs working together in specialised commissioning groups (local specialised commissioning groups for more common specialised services). The planning population for an individual centre is a million people or more.

Out-of-area treatment arrangements cover those situations when someone is admitted to a hospital away from home, usually as an emergency, where there is no pre-arranged service level agreement in place with their PCT. Funding for these ad hoc cases is built into the host PCT's service agreement with their local hospital. Some specialised services activity is excluded from these arrangements.

Teaching PCTs

Teaching PCTs are able to offer GPs and other health professionals clinical posts that involve teaching, research or development. They are not confined to traditional teaching activities such as postgraduate clinical training, continuing professional development and lifelong learning, but aim to provide activities that encompass the ethos of learning, development, research, dissemination and good practice. By offering this type of career development, teaching PCTs hope to attract additional high-quality staff, particularly to deprived areas. Currently 31 PCTs have teaching status.

NHS trusts

There are three main types of NHS trust:

- 176 acute trusts, which provide medical and surgical care and are usually centred on a teaching or district general hospital; an acute trust may manage more than one hospital
- 88 trusts providing mental health services in hospitals or the community
- 32 ambulance trusts.

Some trusts provide a combination of these services, while a few solely manage specialist facilities such as eye or dental hospitals.

NHS trusts earn their income through providing healthcare commissioned by PCTs and set out in a service level agreement between the organisations. They have a legal duty to break even financially, earn a 6 per cent return on their capital and achieve minimum quality standards. They must work in partnership with other NHS organisations, local authorities and the voluntary sector. Trusts are also obliged to deliver national priorities.

Although strategic health authorities manage their performance, trusts are largely self-governing organisations. Their boards comprise a chair, five non-executive directors and five executives – including the chief executive and usually the medical, nursing and finance directors. NHS trusts employ most of the health service's workforce.

Foundation trusts

Foundation trusts are designed to give greater freedoms to NHS organisations, as part of the wider programme of moving from a service controlled nationally to one where standards and inspection are national but delivery and accountability are local.

They are being set up as independent public benefit organisations, modelled on co-operatives and mutual societies, but remain part of the NHS – subject to its standards, performance ratings and inspection systems. Foundation trusts are still accountable to Parliament, but local people have a say in running them by becoming members or governors (see pages 26–7).

An Office of the Regulator authorises and monitors foundation trusts. The office has up to five members and is accountable to Parliament but independent of the health secretary. Its main responsibility is to agree an authorisation with each foundation trust, setting out the framework within which the trust will operate. The Healthcare Commission (see page 56) will inspect foundation trusts, as it does all other NHS organisations.

Foundation trusts' main advantages include:

- increased freedoms to retain any operating surpluses – for example, from land sales – and access to capital from both the public and private sectors; the amount a foundation trust can borrow will be determined by a formula based on its ability to repay the loan, and governed by the prudential borrowing code to be set by the independent regulator
- an obligation to achieve national targets and standards like the rest of the NHS, but freedom to decide how they do this
- not being subject to directions from the Secretary of State
- powers to establish private companies
- the ability to vary staff pay over and above nationally agreed terms and conditions
- not being subject to performance management by strategic health authorities and the DoH.

At present, eligibility for foundation trust status is restricted to NHS trusts with three stars in the performance ratings (see page 59). The first wave of 24 NHS trusts became foundation trusts in April 2004, while another 32 hope to do so from October 2004. The Government's aim is that by 2008 all NHS trusts will have reached a standard suitable for foundation status.

www.dh.gov.uk/PolicyAndGuidance/OrganisationPolicy/SecondaryCare/NHSFoundationTrust/fs/en

Further information
The guide to NHS foundation trusts, DoH, December 2002.

Care trusts

Care trusts are designed to allow close integration of health and social care. They commission and provide both within a single NHS organisation.

The NHS and local authority may establish a care trust together where both agree it offers the best way to improve health and social care. NHS and local authority health-related functions are delegated to the trust, not transferred, and the arrangement is voluntary – partners can withdraw. Local authority councillors are members of the care trust's board. Care trusts may be based on either a primary care trust or an NHS trust.

The concept is intended to be flexible enough to allow for a range of models and service configurations, but care trusts are likely to focus on specialist mental health and older people's services. There are currently eight care trusts.

Children's trusts

The Government's long-term aim, as stated in the 2004 Green Paper *'Every child matters'* is to integrate key children's services within a single organisational focus, the preferred model for which is children's trusts. Most areas should have them by 2006. A children's trust will have the following core features:
- clear short- and long-term objectives
- a children's sevices director in overall charge of delivering these objectives
- a single planning and commissioning function, supported by pooled budgets.

The trust should involve children and families in putting together a picture of their needs and in designing the services to meet those needs through public, private, voluntary and community providers.

Managed clinical networks

Clinical networks are not statutory bodies but partnerships of all organisations and professionals involved in commissioning, planning and providing a particular service in a geographical area. They form, in effect, virtual organisations, and have the potential to break down barriers between primary, secondary and tertiary care and between health and social care. Good working relationships are crucial to their success, and they need multidisciplinary leadership and management.

Networks help ensure all staff with whom a patient has contact are working to the same protocols and policies – for example, on admission, discharge and transfer: this can ease bed shortages and reduce the need for transferring patients between facilities. By collecting all information relevant to a clinical condition they enable network-wide audit to inform practice and future service developments. They encourage staff to work as one on common issues, and share learning.

Networks are now well developed in cancer care, bringing together commissioners and providers, the voluntary sector and local authorities. There are currently 34 cancer care networks, each serving 1 to 2 million people.

Further information

Clinical networks: a discussion paper, NHS Confederation, 2001.

Spotlight on policy: new providers

The Government has declared: 'Working with providers from the independent sector and from overseas is not a temporary measure. They will become a permanent feature of the new NHS landscape and will provide NHS services. Different healthcare providers will work to a common ethos, common standards and a common system of inspection.'

Concordat with the private sector

The NHS Plan noted that a stand-off had existed for decades between the health service and private healthcare providers. Despite this, partnerships between the two had developed, although mostly ad hoc and short-term. As a foundation for a more formal and constructive relationship, the Government drew up a concordat between the NHS and private sector in 2000. Its aim was to enable the NHS to treat more patients more quickly by using spare private healthcare capacity – provided it passed the key test of ensuring high standards of care for the patient and good value for money for the taxpayer.

Spotlight on policy: new providers – *continued*

The concordat covers:

- elective care
- critical care
- intermediate care
- sharing information on workforce planning
- sharing information on service planning.

Organisations agree local protocols for referrals, admissions and discharges between NHS and private facilities. PCTs and trusts can rent accommodation, with elective services delivered by NHS staff, subcontract services to the private sector or commission services from it. They can share information on workforce supply and demand and on adverse clinical incidents. They can also share information about NHS patients treated in the private sector, information necessary for revalidating clinicians and for supporting health improvement planning.

Since the concordat was signed, NHS use of private facilities has increased but remains a small proportion of total activity. Nevertheless, the Government argues that: 'The NHS cannot remain a monolithic, centrally run monopoly provider. Ideological or institutional boundaries should not stand in the way of better care for NHS patients.' As a result, it is now an explicit policy objective to achieve greater plurality in elective surgery services in order to permanently change the nature and increase the volume of services.

Independent sector treatment centres (ISTCs)

The Government is seeking to create units set up and run by independent operators and partly staffed with overseas clinicians. The intention is that ISTCs will make available additional staff, over and above those already working for the NHS, where extra capacity is needed beyond the increase planned by NHS providers. Fifteen companies – including nine from overseas – have been named as qualifying bidders for contracts to provide nine local ISTCs and six chains of centres, one dealing with cataract treatments and five with general diagnostics, surgery and orthopaedic treatments. It is intended they will carry out 135,000 additional operations as well as having 115,000 NHS operations transferred to them. Two are already operational.

The services will be provided in new buildings or refurbished NHS hospitals located in 26 areas; two mobile ophthalmology units will travel to towns across England. NHS staff will work alongside international clinical and managerial teams in the centres.

Spotlight on policy: new providers – *continued*

Overseas clinical teams

The NHS is regularly seeking to attract overseas clinical teams to work in concentrated bursts to supplement capacity in existing organisations, especially in ophthalmics and orthopaedics, where waiting lists have been longest. The scheme aims to use spare capacity in overseas healthcare systems, and seeks to avoid undermining the systems of developing countries. In most cases it is based on short periods of activity – several sessions over a few days or a stay of a few weeks – because the clinical staff continue to practise overseas.

The first teams arrived in 2002, recruited from France, Germany, Italy and South Africa. The DoH is seeking to expand the scope of services overseas that clinical teams can offer.

Overseas treatment for NHS patients

Until recently only about 800 UK patients were treated abroad every year. Most were maternity cases seeking care closer to families in other EU states. But European Court of Justice rulings in 2001 made it clear that UK patients are entitled to receive hospital care in countries in the European Economic Area (the EU, Iceland, Norway and Liechtenstein). Almost 600 patients have taken part in an overseas treatment pilot scheme since 2002, in France, Germany and Belgium, mostly for orthopaedic or cardiac procedures. Reactions have been positive and take-up greater than expected.

There is no earmarked central budget for this, but PCTs must decide on the strength of the case and available options whether to refer patients abroad. They must ensure high quality and value for money, and arrange follow-up care to cope with any complications once patients have returned to the UK. Patients will only travel where that is what they want and after a full clinical assessment shows it meets their needs. Lead commissioning arrangements with Guy's and St Thomas' Trust have been set up to help PCTs wishing to refer patients overseas.

Further information

Growing capacity: a new role for external healthcare providers in England, DoH, June 2002.

The role of boards

Duties and responsibilities

NHS boards take corporate responsibility for their organisation's strategies and actions. They generally consist of five executives (including the chief executive and finance director) and five non-executives plus a chair. The chair and non-executives are lay people drawn from the local community, and are accountable to the Secretary of State.

A board's main duties are:

- collective responsibility for adding value to the organisation by promoting its success through direction and supervision of its affairs
- providing active leadership within a framework of prudent and effective controls which enable risk to be assessed and managed
- setting the organisation's strategic aims, ensuring the necessary financial and human resources are in place for it to meet its objectives and reviewing management performance
- setting and maintaining the organisation's values and standards, while ensuring its obligations to patients, the local community and the Secretary of State are understood and met.

Legally, there is no distinction between the board duties of executive and non-executive directors: they both share responsibility for the organisation's direction and control. The board is expected to bring about change by making best use of all its resources – financial, staffing, physical infrastructure and knowledge – working with staff and partner organisations to meet the public's and patients' expectations. As leaders, board members are expected to understand opportunities for improving services and motivate others to bring them about.

Boards make plans to achieve the Government's objectives for healthcare, guided by the targets and delivery dates in the priorities and planning framework as well as the detailed objectives in the NHS Plan and national service frameworks. Boards have scope to pace their plans to reflect local circumstances, and have a large say over how to achieve them. All boards sign off an annual business plan setting out the year's objectives, and it is the whole board's function to make progress.

NHS boards are obliged to ensure their organisations have an ethos and culture of public service that reflects and respects public expectation. The need for public accountability means boards must conduct business in an open and transparent way that commands public confidence. Their meetings are open to the public, and should be understandable to the public.

Further information

Code of conduct for NHS boards, NHS Confederation.
www.nhsconfed.org/nexus/welcomepack/clinicalgovernance/coc.htm

The chair

As identified by Higgs (see below) and modified to reflect the NHS, the chair's main role is:

- leadership of the board, ensuring its effectiveness in all aspects of its role and setting its agenda
- ensuring provision of accurate, timely and clear information to directors
- ensuring effective communication with staff, patients and the public
- arranging regular evaluation of the board's performance, its committees and individual directors
- helping non-executive directors contribute effectively and ensuring constructive relations between executive and non-executive directors.

Chairs are expected to work up to three days a week. In general, a strong correlation exists between the quality of the chair's and chief executive's leadership and the organisation's success. Where an organisation is not delivering, questions can legitimately be asked about the quality of the board leadership.

Non-executive directors

In 2003 the Higgs Report laid out the responsibilities and expectations of non-executives. Although the report was commissioned by the Department of Trade and Industry and the Treasury to look at commercial enterprises, its principles are relevant to all NHS boards.

Non-executives should:

- constructively challenge and contribute to developing strategy
- scrutinise managers' performance in meeting objectives and monitor the reporting of performance
- satisfy themselves that financial information is accurate and that financial controls and risk management are robust

- be responsible for deciding executive directors' pay, as well as have a prime role in appointing – and where necessary, removing – senior managers and in succession planning
- ensure the board acts in the public's best interests and is fully accountable to it for the organisation's services and the public funds it uses.

The non-executive role is also based on the criteria developed by the NHS Confederation and NHS Appointments Commission, which emphasise the qualities required: steward, ambassador, guardian and experience (SAGE). In practice, boards look for a balance of skills and experience from their non-executives. Some might have professional expertise in accountancy or business management, while others may have experience as a carer or user of the NHS, which may help the board focus its discussions on patient services. But whatever their expertise, all non-executives have a responsibility to engage in all the board's decisions, and should not regard themselves as the person who represents or is interested only in a specific issue.

There are around 4,000 chairs and non-executives on NHS boards. Currently, 48.7 per cent of chairs and non-executives are women – against a goal of 50 per cent – and 12.3 per cent are from ethnic minorities. Although this exceeds the goal of 7 per cent, few are chairs.

The Higgs Report found that private sector non-executives devote between 1.25 and 2.5 days per month to their duties. This compares with the current stipulation of five days for NHS non-executives. Chairs of health authorities and NHS trusts receive up to £20,930 depending on the size of the organisation. PCT chairs get up to £18,608, and all other non-executive directors are paid £5,426 a year.

Further information

Review of the roles and effectiveness of non-executive directors (Higgs Report), DTI, January 2003. www.dti.gov.uk/cld/non_exec_review

Briefing 81: The Higgs Report into the role of non-executive directors, NHS Confederation, May 2003.

For more information on SAGE: www.nhsconfed.org/nexus/welcomepack/sage.htm

The chief executive

The chief executive is responsible for ensuring the board is empowered to govern the organisation and its objectives are accomplished through effective and properly controlled executive action. A chief executive's main responsibilities are:

- leadership
- delivery planning
- performance management
- governance
- accountability.

Board committees

NHS boards may delegate some of their powers to formally constituted committees. Some are set up to advise the board on a permanent basis, such as the:

- audit committee
- remuneration and terms of service committee
- clinical governance committee
- risk management committee.

PCT boards and PECs

Like other NHS organisations, PCTs are overseen by a board consisting of a lay chair and a majority of non-executives, although they must also include a director of public health. In addition, to reflect the importance of clinical leadership in PCTs, each has a professional executive committee (PEC) responsible for its day-to-day running, including developing service policies, investment plans, priorities and projects. This comprises:

- chief executive
- finance director
- at least one social services representative
- a public health professional
- up to 14 healthcare professionals – GPs, nurses, allied health professionals, dentists, pharmacists, optometrists, consultants.

Actual membership is decided locally but must include at least one GP and one nurse. No single profession should be in the majority. The PEC chair is elected by the committee members; the chief executive, finance director and public health professional are ineligible to stand. The PEC chair is automatically a member of the PCT board. A close working relationship between the PEC and the management team led by the chief executive is crucial to a PCT's success.

Foundation trust boards

Foundation trusts are being set up with distinctive governance arrangements to reflect their freedom from central control. Staff, patients and local people are eligible to become 'members' of the trust. Membership entitles them to vote at elections for the board of governors and to stand for election to the board. Members will receive care and treatment at the hospital on exactly the same basis as anyone else.

The board of governors will include those elected by the trust members and staff, as well as people appointed by PCTs and local authorities. Its role will be to advise the board of directors on its forward plans.

Each foundation trust will have a board of directors made up of non-executives appointed by the governors and executive directors appointed by the non-executives, similar to other NHS organisations. This board will be responsible for managing the foundation trust, including its day-to-day operation and forward business plan.

Board of directors meetings will be about the trust's operational business, with board of governors meetings focusing more on members' needs and ensuring local communities can contribute to decision making.

Further information

NHS foundation trusts – a guide to developing governance arrangements, DoH, September 2003.

Key organisation: NHS Appointments Commission

The NHS Appointments Commission makes all chair and non-executive appointments to NHS trusts, PCTs and health authorities. Up to 1,500 people may be appointed annually. The Commission consists of a chair, a chief executive and eight regional commissioners. It has about 55 staff, based in London and Leeds.

Set up as a special health authority following the NHS Plan, the Commission aims to ensure all appointments are made on merit and follow an open, transparent and fair process. Before it existed, health ministers were responsible for appointing all non-executive directors.

The Commission's role does not end once an appointment has been made. Chairs and non-executives look to the regional commissioners for mentoring and support. The Commission, in conjunction with the Leadership Centre, ensures that chairs and non-executives receive proper induction and training in their roles.

Further information

Governing the NHS: a guide for NHS boards, DoH/NHS Appointments Commission, June 2003.

3 Where care is delivered

Primary care

Primary care is where 90 per cent of NHS patients receive their treatment and over 250 million appointments are made every year. Advances in healthcare, especially in diagnostics and minor surgery, mean many more treatments once carried out in hospital can be performed in primary care – a rapidly growing trend convenient for patients and of benefit to the system as a whole. The NHS Plan promised that by December 2004 all patients would be seen by a GP within two working days or by a primary care professional within one working day.

General practitioners

The GP surgery is the focus of most primary care and the source of ever wider-ranging services. In some places, new one-stop primary care centres include GPs, dentists, opticians, health visitors, pharmacists and social workers, bringing into reality a vision of the GP's surgery described in the NHS Plan:

> Many GPs will be working in teams from modern multi-purpose premises alongside nurses, pharmacists, dentists, therapists, opticians, midwives and social care staff. Nurses will have new opportunities, and some GPs will tend to specialise in treating different conditions. The consulting room will become the place where appointments for outpatients and operations are booked, test results received and more diagnosis carried out using video and tele-links to hospital specialists. An increasing number of consultants will take outpatient sessions in local primary care centres.

Practitioners with a special interest

Primary care services are expanding by developing the role of practitioners with special interests.

GPs with a special interest (GPSIs) have additional training and expertise which enables them to provide a clinical service beyond the scope of normal general practice, undertake advanced procedures or develop services. They take referrals from colleagues for conditions in specialities such as ophthalmology, orthopaedics, dermatology and ear, nose and throat surgery, or undertake diagnostic procedures such as endoscopy. GPSIs do not offer a full consultant service, replace consultants or interfere with access to consultants by local GPs. Typically they undertake two sessions a week in their speciality.

GPSIs can increase the capacity of primary care to undertake outpatient appointments, reduce patient waiting times, provide a more convenient service and help to free consultant time in secondary care. Over 1,200 GPSIs are currently practising.

So far, emphasis has been on developing GPs and nurses with special interests, but allied health professionals are now being included.

GMS contract

Most GPs work for the NHS as independent contractors. In 2003, the NHS Confederation on behalf of the DoH negotiated a new general medical services contract which lays down GPs' terms and conditions. It is designed to stop GPs leaving the profession and encourage newly qualified doctors to consider general practice as a career (see page 104).

The GMS contract provides greater scope for collaborative working between practices and across primary care, as well as with secondary care and social services. GPs can choose to provide only essential care for patients who are acutely or chronically ill, or offer a wider range of services, such as contraception, vaccination, minor surgery or the management of complex medical conditions; their pay will be adjusted accordingly. Where GPs opt out of providing out-of-hours care, immunisations, contraception or chronic disease management, PCTs have to find alternative providers.

PMS pilots

GPs can exchange their independent contractor status for a salaried appointment and a personal medical services (PMS) contract. PCTs have found this useful where it has been difficult to recruit and retain GPs under the GMS contract. PMS contract terms are decided between the PCT and GP to tailor services to local needs.

After several successful waves of pilot schemes, PMS has now been made a permanent option. Almost 40 per cent of GPs now work to a PMS contract, compared to 4 per cent when the NHS Plan was published.

Walk-in centres

Walk-in centres provide fast access to advice and treatment for minor ailments and injuries without an appointment. There are now 43 throughout England with expansion planned up to 64. They are open seven days a week, from early morning until late evening, and offer assessment by an experienced NHS nurse as well as information on out-of-hours GP, dental and local pharmacy services.

The centres have seen more than 4 million attendances since they opened in 2000, with an average of 100 a day. As they develop, walk-in centres will offer independent prescribing by nurses and access to GP services so that more patients will receive treatment and prescriptions without having to go to their own practice.

NHS Direct

NHS Direct is a 24-hour telephone health advice and information service staffed by nurses. It provides callers to its helpline (0845 4647) with information on what to do if they or their family are feeling ill, advice on particular health conditions, details of local healthcare services, such as doctors, dentists or late-night pharmacies, as well as self-help and support organisations. Staff use a computer-based decision-support system to suggest the best course of action, and can pass calls directly to emergency services; about 3 per cent of calls are emergencies.

Launched in 1998, NHS Direct handles over half a million calls every month and served its 20 millionth caller in autumn 2003. The top ten symptoms people call about are fever, abdominal pains, vomiting, rash, cough, diarrhoea, headache, cold or flu, toothache and chest pain.

NHS Direct's call-handling capacity will rise from 6 million to 16 million calls annually by 2006, and its phone number will provide a single point of access for out-of-hours care. It will handle all low-priority 999 ambulance calls from 2005.

A special health authority manages the service, and PCTs are responsible for commissioning NHS Direct services.

NHS Direct Online

NHS Direct Online (www.nhsdirect.nhs.uk) is an interactive website that receives over half a million transactions a month. It provides:

- a self-help guide to treating common problems at home
- a 'body key' to identify symptoms
- a health encyclopaedia with over 400 topics

- personal responses to specific requests for information
- a searchable database of hospitals and community health services, GPs, dentists, opticians and pharmacies.

NHS Direct Online information points in public places including hospitals, pharmacies, libraries and supermarkets, provide free access to advice and information using touch screens. More than 500 should be in place by the end of 2004.

The HealthSpace facility offers patients a secure place on NHS Direct Online where, for example, they can record personal health details and make them available to their GP. HealthSpace is being piloted with 8,000 orthopaedic and ophthalmology patients in London during 2004.

NHS Direct Digital TV

An NHS Direct digital TV service will be launched in summer 2004. It will enable users to access health information from their own home at any time. Pilot projects showed that health information on digital TV could reach a wide audience, particularly parts of the population hard to reach through other means.

Over three years, £15 million will be invested in developing and running this interactive service. Initially, information will be provided on:

- NHS services such as directories of GPs, dentists and pharmacies
- an encyclopaedia of illnesses and conditions, tests, treatments and operations
- self-care advice on common health problems
- advice on healthy living
- hot topics on current health issues.

Dental services

Policy on dental services has lagged behind other health sectors. Dentists' commitment to the NHS has waned, leading to problems for many people seeking dental care: four out of ten practices were refusing new patients in 2002. About two-thirds of adults visit their dentist regularly, the rest attending only when they have trouble. Many practices offer a mixture of private and NHS care that can be confusing for patients.

However, PCTs are now to take over funding and commissioning of dental services. They will be able to provide primary dental care themselves or through local contracts. These will cover surgery salaries and expenses instead of the piecework pay system set up when the NHS was founded. Surgeries will be encouraged to broaden their range of services.

An NHS team will support PCTs to tackle long-standing bottlenecks where it is hard to find an NHS dentist. The Dental Practice Board, which deals with fees, will be replaced by a special health authority in 2005.

Community pharmacies

The Government has ambitious plans for the 10,000 high street pharmacies that are visited by 6 million people every day and employ 73 per cent of pharmacists. According to proposals under discussion, they could offer services traditionally only available at GPs' surgeries. The new pharmacy contract, in force from 1 April 2004, aims to improve the range and quality of services of the community pharmacy and integrate it more into the NHS.

Pharmacists could in future:

- advise patients on making best use of prescribed and over-the-counter medicines
- enable patients to get repeat medicines for up to a year without having to contact their GP surgery
- offer longer opening times
- advise on healthy eating, smoking, sexual health.

The Department of Trade and Industry has ruled that PCTs must make it easier for pharmacies to be established in large shopping centres.

Further information

Briefing 93: Community pharmacy, NHS Confederation, December 2003.

Opticians

There are three kinds of registered optician:

Optometrists – or ophthalmic opticians – carry out eye tests, look for signs of eye disease and prescribe and fit glasses and contact lenses. They are graduates who have undertaken a three- or four-year degree in optometry, then spent at least a year in supervised practice before taking professional exams leading to registration with the General Optical Council.

Dispensing opticians fit and sell glasses, and interpret prescriptions, but do not test eyes. Some dispense low-vision aids, and some are qualified to fit contact lenses under instruction from an optometrist.

Ophthalmic medical practitioners are doctors specialising in eyes and eye care. They work to the same terms of service as optometrists.

In addition, ophthalmologists are doctors specialising in eye diseases and most perform eye surgery. They usually work in hospital eye departments. Orthoptists treat disorders of binocular vision, and work in eye departments under the supervision of ophthalmologists. They may also undertake visual screening of children in the community.

Optometrists are independent contractors. Some have specialist skills – for example, in contact lenses, low vision or paediatrics – and can treat patients who would otherwise have to be seen in hospital. Most practices have much of the equipment found in ophthalmology clinics.

Under co-management, or shared care, optometrists working to an agreed protocol undertake specified clinical procedures designed to relieve GPs and the hospital eye service, as well as move patient care into the community. This may cover conditions such as glaucoma, diabetes, cataracts and minor acute eye problems. Optometrists are currently pressing for independent and supplementary prescribing rights.

PCTs are responsible for managing optometrists' contracts. Some employ optometric advisers to provide guidance on issues such as service development, new techniques and treatments, interpreting regulations, investigating complaints and audit.

Community health services

PCTs now provide most community health services. These are services provided in the community by staff such as district nurses, health visitors, podiatrists, speech therapists and physiotherapists. They also include mental health services and services for people with learning disabilities.

Intermediate care

Intermediate care is a vital component of the programme to improve the health and well-being of older people and raise the quality of services they receive. Older people are the main users of the NHS: although they make up about a fifth of the population, they occupy two-thirds of hospital beds, and are three times more likely to be admitted to hospital.

Intermediate care comprises a range of services to promote faster recovery from illness, prevent unnecessary hospital admission, support timely discharge from hospital and maximise a patient's ability to live independently. These services may include:

- rapid-response teams
- hospital-at-home schemes
- supported-discharge teams
- nurse-led facilities in acute or community settings
- council-run or independent residential rehabilitation.

By its nature, intermediate care is not the preserve of any single profession, organisation or sector. It includes health and social care as well as housing, and relies on partnerships between organisations and professions. It has developed enormously in recent years and is on the brink of being recognised as a mainstream service. But as its origins pre-date now established policy directions, intermediate care has evolved in many parts of the country through locally led initiatives in response to local service pressures. This has produced a wide diversity of models.

Secondary care

The changing role of hospitals

Acute hospitals have always dominated healthcare spending and provision. Yet current policy combined with scientific, technological and social developments mean they cannot avoid fundamental change in the next five to ten years. Government pledges to expand the NHS's capacity to improve access to services and offer patients choice mean the NHS must find innovative ways of delivering care and not rely on traditional, hospital-based, solutions. Meanwhile, new financial flows in the system have the potential to shift the balance of power between organisations, stimulating further change.

Many small to medium-sized district general hospitals are experiencing recruitment and retention problems, threatening the viability of some of their services. The European Working Time Directive limiting doctors' hours may make this worse (see pages 108–9). The Royal Colleges and medical school training emphasise the virtues of specialisation, yet many district general hospitals struggle to provide specialists with numbers of appropriate patients adequate to maintain their skills. Until recently, the solution was seen as centralising acute services in large cities, but this has been unpopular with the public, who demand local services. Since medical and technological advances make it possible to carry out more procedures as day cases or in primary care, boundaries between the acute sector and the community will become increasingly blurred.

Key organisation: Independent Reconfiguration Panel

The IRP advises the Secretary of State on proposals for changes to NHS services that have been contested locally. The local authority overview and scrutiny committee may refer a proposal if it is not satisfied:

- with the content of the consultation or the time allowed
- with the reasons given for not carrying out consultation
- that the proposal is in the interests of the health service locally.

The IRP is a last resort when all other options for local resolution have been fully explored. Once a case is accepted for the IRP to consider, the chair agrees any specific terms of reference and a timetable for reporting. The chair will normally appoint a sub-group of three (one health professional, one health manager, one patient and citizen representative) to consider the case. The IRP encourages locally acceptable solutions. Its advice takes account of public and patient involvement and the rigour of local consultation. As a non-departmental public body, the IRP offers advice only: final decisions rest with the Secretary of State.

www.irpanel.org.uk

Treatment centres

Treatment centres promise to be the most powerful and immediate force for change in the acute sector. They are units that carry out planned surgery and treatment, separating them from unplanned care and so lessening the risk that operations have to be cancelled. The Government is counting on them to create innovation, increase productivity and rapidly expand capacity.

A treatment centre's essential features include:

- delivering a high volume of routine treatments and/or diagnostics
- streamlined services using defined pathways
- planned and booked services, with emphasis on patient choice and convenience.

Treatment centres are being developed on various models. Some will be run by the NHS, others by the private sector or overseas providers under contract to the NHS, while others will be public–private partnerships. They may be:

- virtual treatment centres – defined services within an existing hospital, using care pathways to ensure efficiency and enhance the patient's experience
- stand-alone new-build treatment centres – purposely designed for maximum efficiency and to ensure the best patient flows
- refurbished sites – possibly using surplus estate to give quick access to suitable buildings.

The type of work they do falls into three categories:

- short-stay inpatient work, often in a single speciality such as orthopaedics
- day-case or outpatient work, sometimes referred to as 'surgi-centres'
- community-based diagnostic work, such as endoscopy and ultrasound, and minor surgical procedures such as excision of cysts and lesions, and vasectomies.

Centres may serve patients from a limited catchment area or accept those waiting a long time from anywhere. They may care for patients within a single speciality or a range of specialities. There are currently 26 NHS-run treatment centres open, plus two run by the independent sector. The DoH expects 80 to be operational by the end of 2005.

Ambulance services

England's 32 ambulance services made 4 million emergency responses in 2002–03, almost double the number made ten years earlier.

Emergency care is undergoing major changes, driven by a ten-year strategy – Reforming Emergency Care – which calls for faster ambulance response times and better training and equipment for ambulance crews.

Ambulance services respond to 999 calls, doctors' urgent admission requests, high-dependency and inter-hospital transfers, referrals from NHS Direct and major incidents. Emergency calls are prioritised into three categories:

- Category A – which are immediately life-threatening
- Category B or C – which are not life-threatening.

In many areas ambulance trusts also provide transport to get patients to hospital for non-emergency treatment.

Crews now use satellite navigation systems, and soon every emergency ambulance will carry equipment such as ECG machines and telemetry, which lets crews send information about a patient's condition directly to the receiving hospital.

Key organisation: NHS Estates

NHS Estates is a DoH executive agency, providing advice, information and guidance on estates and facilities management. It develops and applies new technologies, promotes advanced designs and design methods and introduces new production techniques, marketing and construction concepts. In particular, it:

- translates professional and technical information for the NHS
- supports trusts in their provision of a warm, safe, comfortable patient environment
- provides support on engineering, decontamination, and the planning, design, procurement and eventual disposal of healthcare buildings
- links estates and facilities management with clinical policy.

It sets national standards for stewardship of the NHS estate, procurement and construction, engineering, design quality and hospitality services. NHS Estates manages a large research and development budget, and has completed projects on, for example, lighting and colour design for hospitals and reducing hospital-acquired infections by design. Work on modernising the estate includes:

- clean hospitals programme – Patient Environment Action Team inspections have ensured no hospitals are now rated poor for cleanliness
- better hospital food – no hospitals are now rated poor
- ward housekeeping – housekeepers are expected to be in place in half of all hospitals by December 2004
- TVs and telephones at the bedside – over 50,000 patients have access
- key worker accommodation – providing affordable housing to help with recruitment and retention of staff.

Its Centre for Healthcare Architecture and Design is dedicated to improving the design of NHS buildings, especially during the service's largest ever construction programme. CHAD employs architects, capital planners and surveyors as well as policy staff.

www.nhsestates.gov.uk

Mental health

Mental illness is as common as asthma, and the costs of treating depression alone are as high as for coronary heart disease. One in four people seek help for a mental health problem at some point in their lives. Mental health is one of the Government's core national priorities (see pages 40–41), with new services and staff being introduced as a result of the NHS Plan.

Organising mental health services

Mental health services are provided as part of primary and secondary care, with responsibility split between the NHS, social services and the voluntary sector. However, PCTs are responsible for commissioning all mental health services. Increasingly PCTs also provide mental health services, often in partnership with a specialist provider. The intention is that this will bring services closer to users, reflect local issues and encourage partnership working across health and social care. There are also 74 specialist mental health trusts which provide acute inpatient care, community and rehabilitation services, residential care centres, day hospitals and drop-in centres. About 80,000 staff work in statutory mental health services.

Primary and community services

About 90 per cent of all patients with mental health problems – including 30 per cent to 50 per cent of all those with serious mental illness – use only primary care services. Nevertheless, 80 per cent of NHS spending on mental health is devoted to inpatient services. Less than half of GPs have postgraduate training in psychiatry and only 2 per cent of practice nurses have mental health training, although about half of GP surgeries provide counselling. GPs refer patients who cannot be helped directly, usually to the local community mental health team (CMHT) or to a psychiatric outpatient clinic.

CMHTs – sometimes known as primary care liaison teams – support most people with mental health problems. They assess and monitor mental health needs using two specialist systems – the care programme approach or care management. These require that everyone seen by specialist mental health services should have their need for treatment assessed, a care plan drawn up and a named mental health worker to co-ordinate their care, including a regular review of their needs. They aim to help provide continuity of care across different services, promote multi-professional and agency working, and ensure appropriate care for people diagnosed with serious mental illness on discharge from hospital.

CMHT members include community psychiatric nurses, social workers, psychologists, occupational therapists, doctors and support workers. Patients will regularly meet the psychiatrist from their mental health team at a psychiatric outpatient clinic for review of their treatment.

Providing mental health services in the community has prompted new approaches to care to avoid hospital admission, such as:

- early intervention teams, which aim to treat psychotic illness as quickly and effectively as possible, especially during the critical period after its onset
- assertive outreach teams to provide intensive support for severely mentally ill people who are difficult to engage in more traditional services
- home treatment and crisis response to provide flexible acute care in patients' own homes with a 24-hour service to help with crises.

Hospital services

Psychiatric hospital services have been progressively scaled down over the last 30 years, as many services once provided in hospitals are now provided in the community. One result of fewer beds and rising demand has been a significant increase in pressure on hospital services, with psychiatric beds experiencing high occupancy rates. Acute inpatient services deal mainly with patients suffering severe mental illness.

Forensic services

Forensic mental health services deal with mentally ill people who may need a degree of physical security and have shown challenging behaviour beyond the scope of general psychiatric services. Some may be mentally disordered offenders.

Services fall into three categories:

- low-security services tend to be based near general psychiatric wards in NHS hospitals
- medium-secure services often operate regionally and usually consist of locked wards with a greater number and a wider range of staff
- high-security services are provided by the three special hospitals (Ashworth, Broadmoor and Rampton), which have much greater levels of security and care for people who pose an immediate and serious risk to others.

In addition, new services are developing to meet the needs of mentally disordered offenders in the community.

Modernising services

The National Service Framework for mental health, published in 1999, sets out a 10-year programme to introduce new standards of care that people will be entitled to expect in every part of the country. It emphasises:

- mental health promotion – to ensure health and social services promote mental health and reduce discrimination and social exclusion associated with mental illness
- primary care and access to services – to deliver better primary mental healthcare and ensure consistent help for people with mental health needs, including primary care services for those with severe mental illness
- effective services for people with severe mental illness – to ensure each person receives the services they need, that crises are anticipated or prevented, that help is prompt and effective if a crisis does occur, and access timely to an appropriate and safe mental health place or hospital bed, as close to home as possible
- caring about carers – to ensure health and social services assess carers' needs and provide care to meet their needs
- preventing suicide – to ensure that health and social services play their full part in reducing the suicide rate by at least one-fifth by 2010.

Revising mental health law

The Government published a draft Mental Health Bill and consultation document in 2002, which proposed reforming the structure and application of mental health law in England and Wales. This was the first major overhaul of the system since the 1950s. The consultation document highlighted the Government's intention to modernise mental health services by:

- increasing investment to make mental health a key priority
- implementing national service frameworks and the NHS Plan, to deliver more effective and accessible support for patients, limiting the need for compulsion
- providing an up-to-date legal framework which promotes patients' rights, protects their safety and public safety.

The bill's aim was to provide a legal structure for requiring mentally disordered people to submit to compulsory treatment, without necessarily requiring them to be detained in hospital – a measure in line with the structure of modern mental health services. It also intended to bring the law more into line with modern human rights law, as defined by the European Convention on Human Rights.

However, by the end of the consultation period there was significant opposition from all key mental health organisations, professionals, carers and users of services. Despite positive aspects, aimed at ensuring care and treatment in the most appropriate setting, more independent judicial decision making and more patient and carer safeguards, it was feared the bill would substantially increase tribunal and expert panel hearings, resulting in more staff being needed. It was also possible the overall number of detentions would increase, through detention of people with personality disorder, compulsory treatment of children and adolescents, and use of community treatment orders.

In November 2003, the Government announced its intention to introduce a revised bill for pre-legislative scrutiny 'as soon as possible'.

In addition, a draft Mental Incapacity Bill was published for consultation in 2003. Its aim is to protect adults who lack mental capacity and help them run their own lives. It creates a new statutory framework for making decisions on behalf of those who lack capacity about financial and welfare matters (including healthcare). A final version is expected in 2004.

Further information

The Draft Mental Health Bill: an assessment of the implications for mental health organisations, NHS Confederation, November 2003.

Involving patients and the public

Involving patients and the public in health services can be interpreted in different ways.

- Individual patients may be involved together with health professionals in making decisions about their own care.
- Users of a particular service may be involved as a group in advising how it might be improved.
- Members of the public may be involved in making strategic decisions about how or where services are to be provided.

The NHS Plan aimed to ensure patients and the public have a real say in how services are planned and developed. The Health and Social Care Act 2001 places a duty on health authorities, primary care trusts and NHS trusts to 'involve and consult' patients and the public. They were already required by law to consult on substantial variations and developments to services; under the act, they must arrange to involve and consult patients and the public in:

- planning services they are responsible for
- developing and considering proposals for changes in the way those services are provided
- decisions to be made that affect how those services operate.

This means discussing with patients and the public their ideas, the organisation's plans, patients' experiences, why services need to change, what people want from services and how to make best use of resources. Boards must consider patient and public involvement issues on their agendas, include among their membership an individual to champion these issues and designate a staff member responsible for the activity. They must commit resources to patient and public involvement, and ensure all staff are trained in it.

The NHS Plan requires every trust to obtain feedback from patients about their experiences of care. In addition, the Healthcare Commission (formerly CHAI, see page 56) is responsible for a programme of national patient surveys (see pages 72–3). Information from patient surveys is used in assessing trusts' performance.

Sweeping reforms to the structure of patient and public involvement have recently taken place, abolishing the community health councils that had existed since 1974 and replacing them with new bodies, outlined below. In addition, local authority overview and scrutiny committees (see page 124) are intended to ensure elected councillors have a say in the NHS in their area, while the public can become members of foundation trusts and elect representatives to the board of governors (see pages 26–7).

Further information

Strengthening accountability: involving patients and the public, DoH, February 2003.

Patient advice and liaison services

Every NHS trust and primary care trust should have a patient advice and liaison service (PALS) providing on-the-spot help and information about health services. PALS aim to:

- resolve concerns before they become major problems
- provide information to patients, carers and their families about local health services and put people in contact with local support groups
- tell people about the complaints procedure and independent complaints advocacy support
- act as an early-warning system by monitoring trends, highlighting gaps in service and making reports for action to trust managers.

Patient and public involvement forums

PPIFs exist for every NHS trust and PCT – 572 in total – in order to influence the day-to-day operation of their services and monitor PALS' effectiveness. They have a minimum of seven members, although the ideal is 15 to 20. It is proposed that PPIFs will have a member appointed as a non-executive director on the trust board. PPIFs' duties include:

- monitoring and reviewing the range and operation of services from the patient's perspective
- seeking patients' views about services
- inspecting NHS premises
- making reports and recommendations to trust managers based on patients' and carers' views and experiences
- referring matters of concern to other NHS bodies or anywhere else they deem appropriate, including the media.

Anyone can apply to be a member. About 140 not-for-profit 'forum support organisations' across England support the PPIFs, under contract to the Commission for Patient and Public Involvement in Health (see overleaf).

DoH director for patients and the public

The Department of Health created a post of director for patients and the public in 2003. The director's role is to:

- champion the voice of patients, carers and the public throughout the NHS and in the DoH
- support staff to work in partnership with patients and carers, and be responsive to their needs
- act as a national spokesperson in promoting and explaining patient-focused policy.

The director reports to the chief nursing officer, who is director of patient experience with board-level responsibility for the DoH's targets to improve patient experience of the NHS.

Key organisation: Commission for Patient and Public Involvment in Health

The CPPIH's remit is to oversee the new system of patient and public involvement, working nationally, regionally and locally to act as a patients' champion. It is an independent, non-departmental public body, sponsored by the DoH.

It sets up, funds and appoints all members to PPIFs, as well as managing their performance. The CPPIH advises the Secretary of State on how the whole system of patient and public involvement is working, and reports on these issues to other national bodies. It also carries out national reviews of services from the patient's perspective – collating data from PPIFs and making recommendations.

The CPPIH's head office is in Birmingham, and it has nine regional centres across England.

www.cppih.org/index.html

Key texts

Kennedy Report
The inquiry into the deaths of child heart patients at Bristol Royal Infirmary from 1984 to 1995 was chaired by Professor Sir Ian Kennedy and made many important recommendations for change in the NHS, not least that there should be representation of patient interests on the inside of the NHS and at every level. It was published in 2001.

www.bristol-inquiry.org.uk

The Expert Patient
This DoH policy document published in 2001 defined a new relationship between patient and professional, in which 'the era of the patient as the passive recipient of healthcare is changing and being replaced by a new emphasis on the relationship between the NHS and the people whom it services'.

Spotlight on policy: patient choice

The NHS has already begun offering choice to people awaiting some surgical procedures, but elective surgery is just a small part of its activity. The Government wants the NHS to deepen and widen the culture of choice, arguing that it is not an end but a means to improving the patient experience. Much debate has concentrated on when and where patients receive treatment, but extending the policy to decisions about what treatments are chosen, and how or whether treatment is given, is a much more radical departure. It will require organisational, cultural and personal changes by organisations, professionals and patients themselves.

The Government wants the service to remain equitable but be responsive to individual needs. Its strategy paper, *Building on the best,* outlines how it wants to see the NHS expand patient choice.

- Patients waiting more than six months for heart surgery are already being offered the chance to have operations in other hospitals within the NHS, in the private sector or abroad. This choice is being extended to other specialities.
- There will be new ways to access primary care, such as nurse-led clinics and polyclinics offering a wide range of GP and specialist services. Diagnostic tests formerly carried out only in hospital will be available here, performed by GPs, nurses and others with specialist interests.
- Commuters will be able to register with a GP near their place of work, instead of at home.
- Patients will be able to get repeat prescriptions for medicines from a pharmacist of their choice for up to a year, without having to go back to their GP. By 2007, new IT arrangements will enable patients to pick up repeat medicines from any pharmacy in England. The range of over-the-counter medicines available without prescription will be expanded, making it easier for patients to manage their own conditions.
- Local services will promote direct access to midwives.
- Patients will be able to enter preferences on to their own electronic care record.

Spotlight on policy: patient choice – *continued*

Giving patients greater choice is a key priority for the NHS. It holds out the prospect of a more responsive service tailored around the individual, with patients as genuine partners in decisions about their care. However, it requires explicit statements about options available to patients, which will involve debate about priorities for investment and the limits to choice. By itself, increased choice may be insufficient to improve the responsiveness of the system – a wider programme of culture change is needed. To ensure equity, policies will need to be targeted at those unable to exercise choice: case managers and advisers to help patients navigate the system will be important in this.

Further information

Building on the best; choice, equity and responsiveness in the NHS, DoH, December 2003.
Patient and public involvement in the NHS: seventh report of session 2002–03, HC697, House of Commons Health Committee, July 2003.

4 NHS strategy: putting policy in context

Joining up the jigsaw of health policy

The NHS has been fundamentally redefined since 1997, moving from a comprehensive system of state funding and public provision to a mixed economy of public, private and voluntary providers – though still state-fund. All current policy initiatives need to be set in this context, where provision will be increasingly pluralistic and diverse.

Alongside this diversity, policies like new funding flows and patient choice could transform the health service as we know it. But there is little appreciation of how these pieces of the health policy jigsaw fit together and their longer-term implications. Each policy strand is discussed in isolation; each has advocates or opponents, but little attempt is made to understand how all the different policies might connect or interact with each other.

Undoubtedly, these new policies could create major changes in the way the NHS works. There are policies that change how patients will use the service, how services are provided and regulated, and a set of enabling policies that support the changes. In addition, there are other changes not under policy-makers' control. Many of the policies are interconnected – for example, developing choice relies on developing the funds flow policy, diversity of provision, regulation, providing information to patients and the IT strategy.

Piecing together the policy jigsaw suggests its diverse elements could bring considerable benefits for patients: improved efficiency and quality; an increased focus on chronic disease management; new types of providers, services and staff more closely matching patient needs; faster and more responsive services; and improved information, giving patients greater control over their care.

However, considerable risks lie ahead: of improvements in efficiency at the expense of quality; the fragmentation of care requiring complex co-ordination; further marginalisation of socially excluded groups and massive changes in local services. The number of major health policy initiatives and the traditional approach of developing and debating them in isolation, mean we do not have a complete understanding of their combined effects on the system.

As yet, policies may not be strong enough to ensure that socially excluded groups and those who do not wish to choose or take control of their care will not be disadvantaged because other users are more adept at using the system.

Unfortunately, the invisible hand of the market does not necessarily force closure or retrenchment on those services that a strategic planning process might have identified as needing to change. The new system may offer incentives for hospitals to increase admissions of less appropriate, lower-severity cases (particularly emergencies) and therefore increase revenues. Often intervention is necessary to correct this. But while there needs to be some sort of strategic oversight, it is important this does not prevent rather than promote change.

Small hospitals have to respond to the centralisation of acute and specialist services and development of new ambulatory care models. Ministers have made it clear they want to shift the debate from closing hospitals to redesigning the services they offer, but the Department of Health has resisted the temptation to provide a masterplan for the pattern of hospital services: health communities, working with local people, will have scope to create locally appropriate models. Removal of some key specialities could lead to the complete collapse of acute services unless some innovative thinking prevents it. Without innovative redesign, traditional hospital organisation is unlikely to be sustainable – not only in rural areas, but in many small and medium-sized towns.

Some elements of the system could hinder needed reform. The governance arrangements for foundation trusts could promote real change by increasing local accountability and giving local stakeholders a greater say in running their hospitals. This would lead to major change in how services are provided. But based as they are on current institutional arrangements, the foundation governance model could also act as a brake on proposals for developing new methods of care delivery that require changes to the nature or size of the institution or integration.

More work needs to be done to forecast the possible effects of the current policy mix and to put in place the requisite organisational development, systems redesign and other measures to deal with potential dysfunctional consequences.

Key text: *The new NHS – modern, dependable*

The Labour Government's first health white paper after coming to power, published in December 1997, announced the setting up of primary care groups (forerunners of PCTs), NICE, CHI and NHS Direct, describing 'a new model for a new century' based on six principles:

- renewing the NHS as a genuinely national service, offering fair access to consistently high-quality, prompt and accessible services across the country
- making delivery of healthcare a local responsibility, with local doctors and nurses shaping services
- getting the NHS to work in partnership, breaking down organisational barriers and forging stronger links with local authorities
- driving efficiency through a more rigorous approach to performance
- shifting the focus on to quality of care to guarantee excellence to all patients, with quality the driving force for decision making at every level
- rebuilding public confidence in the NHS as a public service, accountable to patients, open to the public and shaped by their views.

www.archive.official-documents.co.uk/document/doh/newnhs/newnhs.htm

The planning framework

Public service agreement

Every two years the Treasury conducts a spending review of all Government departments, which covers a three-year span (the third year being carried over to become the first year of the following plan). The Chancellor then announces each department's settlement, and each department draws up a public service agreement (PSA) with the Treasury, setting out what it is expected to provide with its new resources over the three-year period. PSAs are the main way in which the Government tries to ensure that increased resources secure public service reform and improved performance.

The aim of the Department of Health's current PSA is to 'transform the health and social care system so that it produces faster, fairer services that deliver better health and tackle health inequalities'. It sets three objectives, to:

- improve service standards
- improve health and social care outcomes for everyone
- improve value for money.

The Government reported in the 2004 Budget that progress was 'generally excellent', but more remained to be done, including:

- focusing a greater share of NHS resources on public health
- developing a stronger evidence base and putting greater emphasis on prevention
- building on effective joint working between the NHS and social services.

The Chancellor announced in the same Budget that the spending review will respond to the recommendations in the Wanless Report on public health (see pages 89–90) and set out further steps 'to make the delivery of public services more personalised to individual needs'.

Priorities and planning framework

The DoH translates PSA objectives into a priorities and planning framework for the NHS and social services covering three years, so that organisations can look in depth at their services, plan change confidently and implement improvements year on year. Each organisation needs to follow six steps:

- identifying national and local priorities and key targets
- agreeing capacity
- deciding each health and social care organisation's specific responsibilities
- creating robust plans and involving staff and the public in them
- setting up sound arrangements to monitor progress
- improving communication and accountability.

Responsibilities are divided between health and social services. The NHS leads on developing plans for improving access, improving services for cancer, coronary heart disease, improving the patient experience, alleviating health inequalities and drug misuse. Social services lead on improving life chances for children. The NHS and social services lead jointly on mental health and services for older people. Strategic health authorities oversee the planning process and outcome where the NHS is leading, and councils where social services lead. Primary care trusts and councils should agree arrangements where the lead is joint.

Local delivery plans

NHS planning is intended to take place from the bottom up, although within a fairly prescriptive national framework. PCTs develop plans with the help of clinicians as well as patients and the public. There is no longer a formal requirement for PCTs to produce health improvement and modernisation plans (HIMPs), although they are free to develop any plans covering locally agreed priorities not included in the priorities and planning framework.

Each NHS trust creates its own plan; the absence of an acute services strategy makes co-ordinating services difficult. Workforce development confederations (see pages 110–11) work with the other organisations and SHAs to create the workforce plan. SHAs bring together PCT plans to make a comprehensive local delivery plan (LDP), which should cover acute trusts.

The LDP identifies expected progress for each priority area over the three-year planning period, specifying quarterly or annual milestones or even – for a few critical features – planned progress on a month-by-month basis. The LDP is supported by a financial strategy and plan showing how resources are to be deployed and value for money achieved. Although an LDP covers a whole SHA area, it is based on PCT-level plans. It is intended to be a 'live' document that is amended on an ongoing basis if corrective action has to be taken or new initiatives are begun.

The 28 SHA-level LDPs form the basis of the management relationship between the NHS and the DoH. The LDPs show how each area plans to achieve the national targets and key capacity increases. In line with the Government's spending review cycle, plans are completely updated every two years, with year three of the existing plan becoming year one of the new plan.

Key strategy: The NHS Plan

The NHS Plan is the foundation of the Government's reforms for modernising the health service, and links change explicitly to extra investment announced in the March 2000 Budget. Published in July 2000 and intended as an ambitious ten-year programme, the Plan set out to tackle 'systematic problems, which date from 1948 when the NHS was formed'.

Its main features are:

- Funding: will continue to come from taxation, with services free at point of use.
- Facilities: extra beds and equipment, new hospitals and primary care centres, a clean-up campaign for hospitals and 24-hour catering offering better food, modernisation of GP premises.
- Staff: more doctors, nurses and therapists, more training places, better pay and working conditions, including more childcare support.
- Performance: core national standards and targets, independent quality inspection with incentives.
- Partnership: with social services.
- Doctors: new contracts for GPs and consultants.
- Nurses: expanded roles and the introduction of modern matrons and nurse consultants.
- Patients: more information and representation, with increased choice.
- Private sector: concordat to encourage partnerships.
- Waiting times: GP appointments within 48 hours; A&E and other waiting times cut.
- Health inequalities: a national target introduced for reducing inequalities, new screening programmes and smoking cessation services.
- Clinical priorities: major expansion in cancer-screening programmes, rapid access to chest pain clinics, shorter waits for heart operations, new mental health teams.

www.dh.gov.uk

Priorities 2003–06

The current health and social care priorities are:

- improving access to all services through better emergency care, reduced waiting, increased booking for appointments and admission and more choice for patients
- focusing on improving services and outcomes in cancer, coronary heart disease, mental health, older people, improving life chances for children
- improving patients' overall experience
- reducing health inequalities
- contributing to the cross-government drive to reduce drug misuse.

Within each priority area are several key targets, relevant to primary care as well as hospital services and achievable only with close co-operation between health and social services. In addition, local communities have their own priorities, as do local authorities. Nationally, the NHS is looking for significant increases and developments in its physical facilities, workforce and information management and technology.

Work is under way on capacity requirements for 2006–08, which will underpin the 2004 comprehensive spending review, although NHS spending plans until 2008 have already been confirmed.

Key texts

Shifting the balance of power within the NHS

Two documents – *Securing delivery* (July 2001) and *The next steps* (January 2002) – outline the rationale behind devolving power from Whitehall to frontline NHS organisations, in particular PCTs. They announced that SHAs were to replace the existing 95 health authorities and that the DoH would have a reduced role in directly managing the NHS.

Delivering the NHS Plan: next steps on investment, next steps on reform

This document, published in April 2002, introduced plans to reform the NHS's financial flows through payment by results, brought new emphasis to patient choice and underlined commitment to promoting diversity in supply of healthcare through joint ventures with the private sector.

Improvement, expansion and reform: the next three years

This is the NHS's priorities and planning framework for 2003–06. It includes the DoH's public service agreement as an appendix.

5 NHS quality: improving healthcare

Organisations' responsibility for quality

The Government's first health policy white paper, *The new NHS: modern, dependable,* published in 1997, promised that the service 'will have quality at its heart'. NHS organisations now have a statutory duty to ensure the quality of their services, just as they have always had to keep their organisations financially solvent. NHS trust chief executives are accountable for clinical standards, and each trust has a designated senior clinician who must make sure clinical governance systems are functioning properly. Primary care trusts have to nominate a senior health professional, usually a GP, to lead on clinical standards and professional development. In essence, NHS organisations must:

- develop an open and participative culture
- demonstrate a commitment to quality
- work routinely with patients, users, carers and the public
- encourage an ethos of multidisciplinary team-working at all levels
- reduce unjustifiable variations in quality of care
- share good practice
- detect and deal with poor performance and adverse events.

The Government's aim is to provide clear, national standards for services supported by consistent evidence-based guidance to raise quality, and to put in place a robust system of inspection. It wants to see:

- continuous improvement in quality of care
- a reduction in unacceptable variations in clinical practice
- best use of resources so that patients receive maximum benefit.

Research has found that, in general, patients expect a high-quality health service to provide:

- treatment that is effective and delivers good outcomes
- services that are quick and easy to use
- services that are well organised
- treatment with dignity and respect
- treatment in places that are safe.

Clinical governance

Clinical governance is an explicit framework for making all NHS staff accountable for quality improvement and safeguarding standards, ensuring that quality remains a priority. The chief medical officer's definition of clinical governance is:

> a system through which NHS organisations are accountable for continuously improving the quality of their services and safeguarding high standards of care, by creating an environment in which clinical excellence will flourish.

It seeks to transform the culture, ways of working and systems of every health organisation so that patient safety, quality assurance and improvement are an integral part of their everyday work. Its main features are a coherent approach to quality improvement, clear lines of accountability for clinical quality systems and effective processes for identifying and managing risk and addressing poor performance.

Its essential components are:

- the patient's experience – of access to services, organisation of care, the humanity of care and the environment in which care is delivered
- the organisation's use of information
- consultation and patient involvement
- risk management
- clinical audit
- effectiveness and research
- staffing and staff management
- education, training and continuing professional development
- leadership
- direction and planning, accountability and structures
- partnership with the public
- partnership with the local health economy.

For clinical governance to work properly and quality to flourish, NHS organisations must foster a culture of openness and participation, value education and research, and encourage people to learn from failures. Good practice and new approaches should be shared readily and received willingly.

Key organisation: The Healthcare Commission

The Commission's role is to independently assess standards of patient services, whether provided by the NHS or privately. It is independent of the Government and reports to Parliament.

The Healthcare Commission, known as the Commission for Healthcare Audit before its launch, has taken over the functions of:
- the Commission for Health Improvement
- the National Care Standards Commission, responsible for inspecting private and voluntary healthcare
- the Audit Commission, in respect of national studies into the efficiency, effectiveness and economy of healthcare.

In due course, the Commission is expected to take over the functions of the Mental Health Act Commission.

It will also have new functions:
- independently assessing complaints
- assessing the arrangements in place to promote public health
- acting as the leading inspectorate in relation to healthcare.

It will inspect arrangements for clinical governance in local NHS organisations, as well as register, inspect and regulate independent healthcare providers. It will publish the annual star ratings for NHS organisations, and co-ordinate the activity of other bodies involved in inspecting healthcare establishments.

The Government has stated that the Commission's underlying purposes are to:
- provide patients with clear assessments of the safety, quality, efficiency and effectiveness of services
- maximise the contribution which regulation may make to improving health and social services
- reduce the burden of regulation on providers of health and social services.

www.healthcarecommission.org.uk

National service frameworks

National service frameworks (NSFs) are evidence-based programmes setting quality standards and specifying services that should be available for a particular condition or care group across the whole NHS. They are intended to eradicate local variations in standards and services, raise standards generally, promote collaboration between organisations and contribute to improving public health. Each identifies key interventions, puts in place a strategy to support implementation and establishes an agreed timescale.

Each NSF is developed with assistance from an external reference group of health professionals, service users and carers, health service managers, partner agencies and other advocates. The DoH supports the groups and manages the overall process.

Usually only one new NSF is released in a year. The programme, begun in 1998, so far covers:

- mental health, September 1999 (see page 40)
- coronary heart disease, March 2000
- cancer, September 2000
- older people, March 2001
- diabetes: standards, December 2001; delivery strategy, January 2003
- renal services: part one, January 2004
- long-term conditions, late 2004
- children: hospital standards, April 2003; remainder 2004.

Collaboratives

Collaboratives have been used widely in the NHS to improve service quality. They are structured, time-limited programmes focusing on a specific topic. They offer clinical and management teams opportunities to learn new tools and techniques and share practices to improve the quality and provision of care. The method has proven effective in primary care – where over 2,000 practices have taken part – for cancer, coronary heart disease (involving 30 local CHD programmes) and emergency services, as well as in other national healthcare systems.

Performance assessment in transition

The Government has acknowledged that the standards against which healthcare has been measured have formed 'a complex multiplicity, often seemingly random, and they can be bewildering and frustrating to busy clinicians'. NHS performance assessment is therefore in transition. Changes are under way aimed at eradicating the unco-ordinated nature of the system and replacing it with a framework that will help the Healthcare Commission in its inspections, as well as provide patients and the public with an assurance of what they can expect from the NHS.

Standards for better health

Existing targets will be replaced with 'key standards' in two categories: core and developmental. The 24 core standards will establish a level of quality that all NHS patients can expect, regardless of where they are treated. The ten developmental standards are designed to enable overall healthcare quality to rise as additional resources take effect, reflecting new healthcare trends and public attitudes to the service. Together they address the seven 'domains' of NHS healthcare:

- safety
- clinical and cost effectiveness
- governance
- patient focus
- accessible and responsive care
- care environment and amenities
- public health.

The Government believes that fewer centrally-specified targets will be needed in an NHS where money follows patients and services are driven by their preferences while more power is devolved to frontline staff.

However, the Healthcare Commission, as the independent regulator, is responsible for developing the ratings system and the way in which trusts' ratings are calculated. It will be the Commission's role to decide how many criteria to attach to each standard and develop the methodology for measuring it. The Commission has said star ratings could be abolished from 2006 and replaced by richer data on 'relative performance' rather than a 'succeed or fail approach', although the Government has insisted star ratings will continue.

Further information

Standards for Better Health: health care standards for services under the NHS – a consultation, DoH, February 2004.
Briefing 95: Standards for better health, NHS Confederation, March 2004.

Performance assessment framework

The national performance assessment framework rests on six high-level indicators focusing on quality and efficiency and designed to provide a 'balanced scorecard' against which to measure NHS performance in the round. The framework is also intended to encourage benchmarking between similar organisations and underpin accountability arrangements locally and nationally. The six indicators are interdependent and are shown in the diagram opposite.

The elements of the performance assessment framework

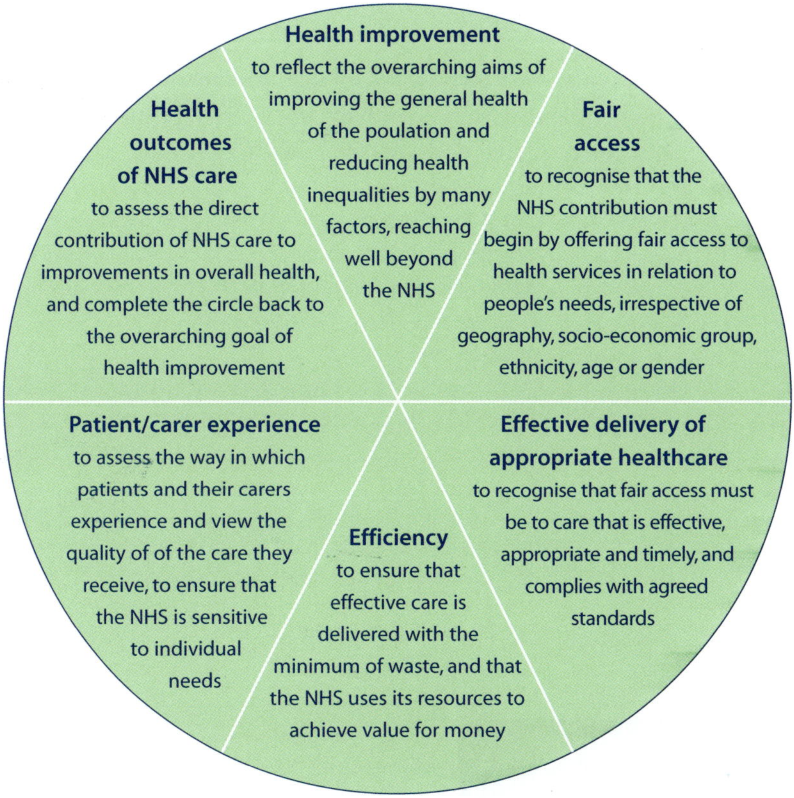

Star ratings

Performance ratings for acute, specialist, mental health and ambulance trusts, and for primary care trusts, are published annually. Each organisation is awarded stars for its performance. This system is intended to provide NHS staff and the public with accessible and easy-to-understand information about the performance of local health services. The ratings tables allow trusts to compare their performance against others, so they can share good practice and address weaknesses.

The star rating system places trusts into one of four categories:

- *Three-star trusts* demonstrate the highest level of performance and are rewarded with more capital and fewer central reporting requirements and inspections. Only three-star trusts can apply for foundation status. They also enjoy other benefits from earned autonomy.
- *Two-star trusts* are performing well overall across the range of indicators, but need to improve in particular areas. They are subject to normal reporting arrangements, but enjoy higher delegated limits for approving capital investments and freedom to retain more of the proceeds of local land sales.
- *One-star trusts* give some cause for concern against particular key targets and are subject to much closer oversight by their SHA, which will develop improvement plans. Occasionally key personnel will be seconded to the trust – for example, at chief executive level – to drive forward improvements, and the Modernisation Agency will be closely involved.
- *Zero-star trusts* show the poorest levels of performance against key targets, and are required to produce performance improvement plans within three months to demonstrate how they intend to turn the organisation around. In some cases they are subject to franchising.

Star ratings for 2002–03: overall results for NHS trusts and PCTs

3 stars	–	133
2 stars	–	257
1 star	–	165
0 stars	–	44

Source: CHI

The Government intends that by 2008 all NHS hospitals will consistently perform sufficiently well to become foundation trusts. Its improvement programme, aimed at two-, one- and zero-star trusts and PCTs, provides:

- a clear assessment of the organisation's needs
- tailored support from the Modernisation Agency and others
- leadership development
- targeted resources.

The future

The DoH is consulting on changes to the performance assessment system which would replace existing targets with 'key standards' in two categories: core and developmental. The 24 core standards would establish a level of quality that all NHS patients could expect, regardless of where they were treated. The ten developmental standards are designed to enable overall healthcare quality to rise as additional resources take effect, reflecting new healthcare trends and public attitudes to the service. Together they address the seven 'domains' of NHS healthcare:

- safety
- clinical and cost effectiveness
- governance
- patient focus
- accessible and responsive care
- care environment and amenities
- public health.

In theory, the Government believes, fewer centrally specified targets will be needed in an NHS where money follows patients and services are driven by their preferences while more power is devolved to frontline staff.

However, the Healthcare Commission (formerly CHAI), as the independent regulator, is responsible for developing the ratings system and the way in which trusts' ratings are calculated. It will be the Commission's role to decide how many criteria to attach to each standard and develop the methodology for measuring it. The Commission has said star ratings could be abolished from 2006 and replaced by richer data on 'relative performance' rather than a 'succeed or fail approach', although the Government has insisted star ratings will continue.

Further information

Standards for better health: health care standards for services under the NHS – a consultation, DoH, February 2004.

Briefing 95: Standards for better health, NHS Confederation, March 2004.

Earned autonomy and franchising

The concept of earned autonomy, established in the NHS Plan, rewards organisations which perform well. The more an organisation's performance improves, the greater its freedom to manage its own affairs. Specifically, three-star trusts benefit from:

- higher delegated limits for the approval of capital investments
- retention of more proceeds from local land sales for reinvestment in services
- opportunities to shape national policy
- less frequent monitoring from the centre
- removal of management cost limits (PCTs do not have limits)
- automatic entry on the NHS Franchising Register of Expertise
- additional freedom when establishing spin-off companies
- being used as pilot sites for new initiatives
- additional funding for sabbaticals and staff exchanges where a trust has released staff to support other NHS organisations or DoH policy work
- a more hands-off relationship with the SHA.

For a failing trust, the last resort in 'extreme cases of under-performance' is to franchise its management, usually to experienced NHS managers with a proven track record. Where the SHA considers the organisation has insufficient capacity to improve, it will consult ministers on whether to franchise. The NHS Franchising Register of Expertise includes more than 70 organisations able to tender for franchises to manage poorly performing trusts. It automatically includes three-star trusts, and currently lists eight private companies.

Key organisation: National Institute for Clinical Excellence (NICE)

NICE is a special health authority set up in 1999 to provide guidance for professionals, managers, patients and carers on decisions about treatment and healthcare. Currently this covers:

- technology appraisals
- clinical guidelines
- the use of new surgical (or other interventional) procedures.

Technology appraisals are independent reviews of the clinical and economic evidence on the appropriate use of specific technologies, such as medicines, medical devices, diagnostic techniques, surgical procedures and health promotion activities.

Key organisation: National Institute for Clinical Excellence (NICE) – *continued*

Clinical guidelines provide recommendations on the appropriate NHS treatment and care of patients with specific diseases and conditions. NICE has established seven national collaborating centres to harness the expertise of the Royal Colleges and patient/carer organisations when developing clinical guidelines. These cover acute care, cancer, chronic conditions, mental health, nursing and supportive care, primary care and women's and children's health.

Topics for technology appraisals and clinical guidelines are referred to NICE by the Secretary of State for Health. Proposals can come from horizon scanning of clinical innovations, special mapping exercises in particular clinical areas, patients and carers, patient groups, professionals, NHS organisations and industry. Each year NICE develops around 25 technology appraisals and ten clinical guidelines.

Its 30-strong citizens council keeps NICE informed on what the public thinks about the use of treatments and NHS care. Members are drawn from all age groups, social circumstances, ethnic backgrounds, regions and abilities. They meet in public twice a year for three-day sessions to debate questions put to them by the NICE board.

The NHS has to provide funding for treatments and drugs recommended by the NICE technology appraisal process. Although NICE guidance does not override the responsibility of healthcare professionals to make appropriate decisions based on the circumstances of individual patients, they are expected to take it fully into account when exercising clinical judgement. NICE guidance recommendations are prepared by independent teams of experts, which include healthcare professionals and lay people. These guideline development groups and advisory committees seek the views of organisations representing healthcare professionals, patient and carers, manufacturers and Government, but their advice is independent of any vested interests. NICE also has a partners council with members drawn from the key organisations representing patients and carers, healthcare professions and NHS managers. The council advises NICE on key strategic issues and reviews its annual report.

NICE also funds three organisations that undertake research into the way patients are treated. These National Confidential Enquiries cover suicide and homicide, maternal and child health, and patient outcome and death.

www.nice.org.uk

Reforming clinical negligence procedures

Although the NHS provides high-quality healthcare for millions of people every year, occasionally patients do not receive the treatment they should, or mistakes are made. About 10 per cent of hospital inpatient admissions may result in some kind of adverse event, while 5 per cent of the population report suffering some injury or other adverse effects of medical care; almost a third of those claim it had a permanent impact on their health. About 18 per cent of patients say they suffered a medication error some time in the previous two years.

Anyone who suffers harm as a result of treatment must receive an apology, a clear explanation of what went wrong, proper treatment and care and, where appropriate, financial compensation. The NHS must ensure it learns from such experiences.

However, legal proceedings for medical injury frequently involve confrontation, revealing as little as possible about what went wrong, defending clinical decisions and only reluctantly releasing information. The process has proved complex, has been sometimes unfair and almost always slow and expensive, with legal costs exceeding compensation awards in many cases. After consultation, the chief medical officer therefore published in 2003 proposals for reforming NHS clinical negligence procedures.

The proposals aim to ensure the NHS strives to prevent harm, reduce risks and enhance safety. They are designed to encourage a better co-ordinated response to harm, including investigation, support, remedial treatment and care and fair recompense. The system of redress should be affordable and reasonably predictable in the way it operates, as well as act as an incentive to NHS organisations and staff to improve quality of care and patient safety.

The main proposal is for an NHS Redress Scheme to provide:

- investigations when things go wrong
- remedial treatment, rehabilitation and care
- explanations and apologies
- financial compensation in certain circumstances.

It would also provide care and compensation for severely neurologically impaired babies, including those with severe cerebral palsy where their impairment was birth-related. A national body, building on the NHS Litigation Authority's work, is likely to oversee the scheme and manage the financial compensation nationally. Patients or families who chose not to apply for packages of care and payment under the scheme would still have the right to pursue litigation, although those who did accept a package under the scheme would not be able to sue for the same injury through the courts. Every trust would appoint someone at board level to take overall responsibility for investigating and learning from adverse events, complaints and claims.

Key organisations

National Patient Safety Agency

The NPSA aims to harness systematic learning from patient safety incidents and service failure in the NHS, collecting and analysing information from local NHS organisations, staff, patients and carers, and initiating preventive measures so that the whole service can learn from each case. It ensures that where risks are identified, work is undertaken on solutions, and it specifies national goals and mechanisms to track progress. As well as making sure that incidents are reported, the NPSA aims to promote an open and fair culture across the health service, encouraging staff to report incidents and near-misses.

www.npsa.nhs.uk

NHS Litigation Authority

The NHSLA indemnifies NHS bodies against clinical negligence and non-clinical risks, and manages claims and litigation covering both. It has a panel of 13 specialist firms of solicitors which are instructed on clinical negligence claims. In 2002–03 it received 7,798 claims for clinical negligence and had potential liabilities for clinical negligence of £5.9 billion.

www.nhsla.com

Key texts

A first class service: quality in the new NHS

Published in June 1998, this provides the blueprint for ensuring quality. Its main themes are the importance of national consistency in implementing evidence-based practice, accountability for local best practice, commitment to a coherent system of quality improvement and assurance, provision for managing poor performance and professional collaboration and teamwork.

An organisation with a memory

Compiled by an expert group led by the chief medical officer and published in June 2000, this recommended a mandatory reporting scheme for adverse healthcare events and near-misses. It set out to encourage a reporting and questioning culture in the NHS to replace blame with a proper understanding of the underlying causes of failures.

Making amends

This sets out 19 proposals for consultation intended to fundamentally reform the handling of clinical negligence cases, including establishment of an NHS redress scheme to speed up the process and offer care and compensation without going to court. It was published in June 2003.

Healthcare professions' responsibility for quality

Modernising professional self-regulation

NHS patients need to know that the staff who care for them are well-trained and competent. Professional self-regulation has been a cornerstone of the NHS since it began, yet events such as the Bristol Inquiry and the Alder Hey cases – in which organs from dead children were retained without their families' knowledge – highlighted the need for reform.

Professional self-regulation covers education, registration, training, continuing professional development and revalidation. It includes setting standards for deciding who should enter and remain members of a profession, and determining their fitness to practise. Its underpinning principles are:

- clarity about standards
- maintaining public confidence
- transparency in tackling fitness to practise
- responsiveness to and protection of patients.

The NHS Plan stipulated that regulatory bodies had to reform to become smaller, with much greater public and patient representation, faster, more transparent procedures and more meaningful accountability to the public and the health service. This was reinforced by the Kennedy Report on the Bristol Royal Infirmary inquiry a year later (see page 44). The Government has insisted that regulators develop common systems across the professions and agree standards that put patients' interests first. It is keen that self-regulation keeps pace with change in the NHS as well as society's attitudes and public opinion. Professional regulatory bodies must be open and make improvements based on feedback from patients, their representatives and the public. They must deal with complaints quickly, thoroughly, objectively and in a way that is responsive to the complainant while treating fairly the health professional complained against.

New regulatory bodies have been introduced for nursing, midwifery and health visiting and for the allied health professions:

- The Nursing and Midwifery Council replaced the UK Central Council in 2002 as the body responsible for governing nurses, midwives and health visitors.
- The Health Professions Council is responsible for the professions previously regulated by the Council for Professions Supplementary to Medicine, and includes groups of healthcare professionals not previously covered by formal statutory regulation.
- The Council for the Regulation of Healthcare Professionals (see overleaf) oversees all the other professional regulatory bodies.

Legislation has changed the General Medical Council's make up and lines of accountability, reformed its fitness-to-practise procedures and introduced revalidation for all doctors.

In March 2004 the Government opened a consultation on proposals to extend regulation to all healthcare staff whose work has a direct impact on patient clinical care. www.dh.gov.uk/Consultations/fs/en

Further information

Supporting doctors, protecting patients: a consultation paper on preventing, recognising and dealing with poor clinical performance of doctors in the NHS in England, DoH, 1999.
General Medical Council: www.gmc-uk.org
Nursing and Midwifery Council: www.nmc-uk.org
Health Professions Council: www.hpc-uk.org

Key organisation: Council for the Regulation of Health Care Professionals

CRHP is a statutory body responsible to Parliament and independent of the Department of Health. It promotes best practice and consistency in professional self-regulation in nine bodies:

- General Medical Council
- General Dental Council
- General Optical Council
- General Osteopathic Council
- General Chiropractic Council
- Health Professions Council
- Nursing and Midwifery Council
- Royal Pharmaceutical Society of Great Britain
- Pharmaceutical Society of Northern Ireland.

It has 19 members – one from each of the nine bodies and ten lay members. With parliamentary approval, CRHP can force a regulator to change its rules. It also has the power to refer unduly lenient decisions about professionals' fitness to practise to the High Court for review.

www.crhp.org.uk

Continuing professional development

In *A first class service* (see page 66), the DoH defined continuing professional development (CPD) as:

> a process of lifelong learning for all individuals and teams which meets the needs of patients and delivers the health outcomes and healthcare priorities of the NHS, and which enables professionals to expand and fulfil their potential.

In a climate of constant change, it is important that members of all professions demonstrate that they are keeping their knowledge and skills up to date: it is no longer sufficient simply to establish competence at the beginning of a career. Many professions, not just in healthcare, are beginning to adopt mandatory CPD. For individuals, CPD should:

- maintain professional competence and enable them, their teams and organisation to meet patients' needs, carry out their work with confidence and assist them in the event of an untoward incident

- provide them with the professional and personal satisfaction that they are working to the best of their ability and for the greater benefit of patients, colleagues and their employer
- help sustain motivation and interest in their work
- help meet career aspirations and learning needs, support flexible career pathways and allow them to take on wider responsibilities if necessary
- help them keep their jobs or enhance the possibility of finding another job
- help them identify the skills and knowledge they need to develop, preparing them for future opportunities.

CPD is a cyclical process involving four components:

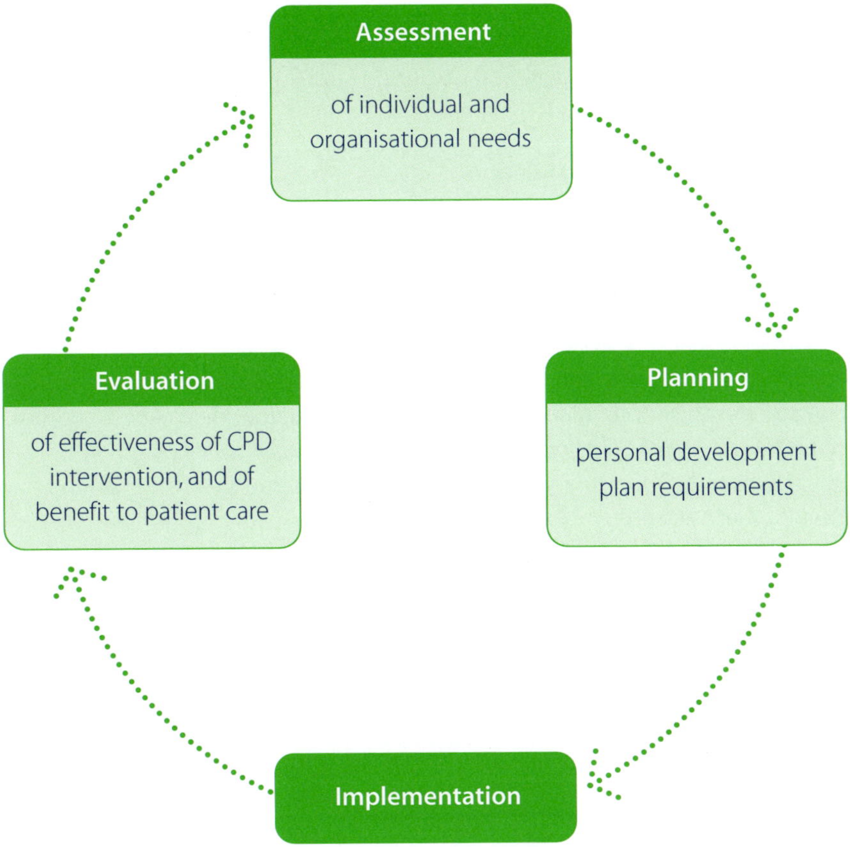

CPD is as important for NHS organisations as it is for individuals. A professional's failure to keep up to date could have serious results, while allowing their skills and knowledge to become obsolete is to waste the investment in their education and training. In *Continuing professional development – quality in the new NHS* (July 1999) the DoH stated that 'every health organisation needs to develop a locally managed, systematic approach to CPD'. The core principles are that CPD should be:

- purposeful and patient-centred
- participative, fully involving the individual and other relevant stakeholders
- targeted at identified educational need
- educationally effective
- part of a wider organisational development plan supporting local and national service objectives
- focused on the development needs of clinical teams across traditional professional and service boundaries
- designed to build on previous knowledge, skills and experience
- designed to enhance the skills of interpreting and applying knowledge based on research and development.

Doctors' appraisal and revalidation

Appraisal systems are now in place for all the major groups of NHS doctors, developed jointly by the DoH, British Medical Association (BMA) and the General Medical Council (GMC) to give doctors regular feedback on past performance and continuing progress. The aims are to:

- set out personal and professional development needs, career paths and goals
- agree plans for them to be met, and review the doctor's performance regularly
- consider the doctor's contribution to the quality and improvement of local healthcare
- optimise the use of skills and resources to achieve high-quality care
- offer doctors an opportunity to discuss and seek support for taking part in development activities
- identify the need for adequate resources to enable service objectives to be met.

Appraisal is based on the GMC's document, *Good medical practice*, which describes the standards of competence, care and conduct expected of doctors. These are:

- good clinical care
- maintaining good medical practice
- teaching and training
- relationships with patients
- working with colleagues
- probity
- health.

Appraisal should include data on clinical performance, training and education, audit, concerns raised and serious clinical complaints, application of relevant clinical guidelines, relationships with patients and colleagues, teaching and research activities, and personal and organisational effectiveness. Every doctor undergoing appraisal needs to prepare a folder of information, evidence and data.

The appraiser should have a good understanding of the doctor's work. Doctor and appraiser agree a written summary of the appraisal, outlining achievement in the previous year, objectives for the next year, key elements of a personal development plan, actions expected of the organisation, and a joint declaration that the appraisal has been carried out properly. Chief executives of NHS organisations are responsible for ensuring appraisals take place and that appraisers are properly trained.

Appraisal and revalidation are two separate processes with different objectives but are based on the same sources of information, and the outcome of an individual's appraisal will be used for revalidation.

The GMC says it will grant doctors a licence to practise by the end of 2004 unless they tell the GMC they don't want one. If a doctor is not on the Medical Register by the end of 2004, they will get a licence automatically when they are registered. To maintain a licence to practise, doctors must take part in revalidation when the GMC asks them. The GMC will start to invite doctors for revalidation in spring 2005.

Further information

www.appraisaluk.info
www.revalidationuk.info

Key organisation: National Clinical Assessment Authority

The NCAA helps NHS organisations deal with doctors and dentists whose performance causes concern. It takes referrals and provides advice about handling cases locally, carrying out its own clinical performance assessments where necessary and recommending solutions. These may involve retraining, disciplining or suspending doctors whose practice causes serious concern. The NCAA is an advisory body, and the NHS employer organisation remains responsible for resolving the problem once the NCAA has produced its assessment.

www.ncaa.nhs.uk

Code of conduct for NHS managers

Just as doctors, nurses and other health workers have codified ethics, so now do NHS managers. Written by senior managers in collaboration with the DoH, the code states that all NHS managers must:

- make the care and safety of patients their first concern and act to protect them from risk
- respect the public, patients, relatives, carers, NHS staff and partners in other agencies
- be honest and act with integrity
- accept responsibility for their own work and the proper performance of the people they manage
- show their commitment to working as a team member by working with all their colleagues in the NHS and the wider community
- take responsibility for their own learning and development.

NHS organisations must incorporate the code in the contracts of chief executives and directors, and investigate alleged breaches. Those who break the code can be dismissed from the NHS and barred from re-employment within it.

Further information

Briefing 78: Managing for excellence in the NHS and the code of conduct for NHS managers, NHS Confederation, February 2003.
www.nhsconfed.org/connecting/code_of_practice.asp

Feedback from patients

National patient surveys

Listening to patients' views is essential for a patient-centred health service. To deliver improvements, the NHS has to know what people need and expect from it, and how well they think the service has responded to their needs and expectations.

The Government proposed introducing surveys of patients and health service users in *The new NHS: modern, dependable* and repeated the commitment in the NHS Plan. The programme of national patient surveys has three aims:

- to provide feedback for local quality improvement
- to assess users' experience for performance ratings, inspections and reviews
- to monitor patients' experience nationally.

The Healthcare Commission (formerly CHAI) has taken on the responsibility for carrying out national survey programmes (previously handled by the Commission for Health Improvement). In 2003, over 59,000 patients in 155 NHS trusts were involved in the acute trusts' emergency department survey, and over 90,000 patients in 171 trusts in the outpatient survey. Over 123,000 patients in 304 primary care trusts were involved in the PCT patient survey. The results were grouped into five areas:

- access and waiting
- information and choice
- building relationships
- cleanliness, comfort and friendliness
- safety, quality and co-ordination of care.

Several surveys are taking place during 2004:

- adult inpatients in acute and specialist trusts
- young patients (inpatients and day-cases under 18) in acute and specialist trusts
- PCT survey (people 16 years and over)
- mental health service users (adults of working age on the care programme approach)
- ambulance trusts (urgent and emergency cases)
- national service framework surveys on coronary heart disease and stroke patients.

Local patient surveys

The NHS Plan also requires each trust to obtain feedback from its own patients about their experiences of care. These surveys are intended to:

- track changes in patients' experience at trusts, year on year
- provide information for local quality improvement initiatives
- inform each trust's performance ratings and the performance indicators.

Trusts can seek support in carrying out their surveys from the NHS Patient Survey Programme Advice Centre.

Further information

NHS Patient Survey Programme Advice Centre: www.nhssurveys.org

Complaints

Reforming the system

The Government has published proposals for reforming the current NHS complaints procedure – which dates from 1996 – to make it more independent and responsive to patients' needs. Patients were found to be particularly dissatisfied with the independent review stage, which they perceived not to be truly independent or impartial. The evaluation found that 'improving this aspect of the current procedure is the single most commonly cited suggestion for reform'.

The proposed changes cover all services provided by NHS trusts (including foundation trusts) primary care trusts, primary care practitioners, strategic health authorities and most special health authorities. Independent sector organisations providing care for the NHS will, through their contracts, have to operate a comparable complaints process.

Under the proposed changes, the essential structure remains the same. Complaints are received and responded to locally; if resolution is not achieved, there is an independent review of the complaint; and if the complainant remains unhappy, they may involve the Ombudsman. But a number of changes are designed to link the procedure more closely to systems for improving services:

- The Healthcare Commission (formerly CHAI) will independently review complaints when complainants are unhappy with the local response. This will involve an investigation by Commission staff and, if appropriate, by a panel of lay people.
- People can complain about primary care services either directly to the practitioner or to the PCT.
- Complaints may be raised with any staff member and resolved on the spot. They need not be dealt with more formally than that unless the complainant wishes it. A complaint may be about any matter connected with the NHS's services, including decisions that affect people who are neither current nor former patients – often to do with access to services.
- The time limit for making a complaint will be extended from six months to one year. Complaints should be acknowledged within two working days, and responded to in 25 working days – unless the complaint is complex and provided a longer response time is acceptable to the complainant. A complaint that has not been resolved within six months may be referred to The Healthcare Commission.
- NHS organisations and primary care practitioners have a new duty to co-operate in receiving and investigating complaints, and providing single and comprehensive responses to complainants.
- They must designate a board member or similarly senior person to ensure that complainants receive full consideration and responses, and that action is taken as a result of investigations. Regular reports are required on the numbers of complaints received, the substance of those complaints and the action taken as a result.

Further information

NHS complaints reform – making things right, DoH, December 2003

Independent Complaints Advocacy Services (ICAS)

Every trust and PCT will have an ICAS to help individuals pursue complaints about the NHS. Complainants can contact their local ICAS office direct, or through complaints managers at hospitals and GP practices, NHS Direct, or the patient advice and liaison service. ICAS aims to ensure complainants have access to the support they need to articulate their concerns and navigate the complaints system. It can simply offer advice or write letters and attend meetings to speak on the complainant's behalf.

The Commission for Patient and Public Involvement in Health (see page 44) sets standards for ICAS, while PCT patient forums will be responsible for commissioning local ICAS.

Key organisation: the Ombudsman

The office of the Parliamentary and Health Service Ombudsman (sometimes referred to as the Health Service Commissioner) undertakes independent investigations into complaints about the NHS, as well as Government departments and other public bodies. It is completely independent of the NHS and Government. In the NHS, the Ombudsman investigates complaints that a hardship or injustice has been caused by its failure to provide a service, by a failure in service or by maladministration. The Ombudsman looks into complaints against private health providers only if the treatment was funded by the NHS.

Complainants can only refer their cases to the Ombudsman after failing to achieve a resolution with the organisation or practitioner they are complaining against – for example, because of delays in dealing with a complaint locally, an unreasonable refusal to convene an independent panel review, or failure to get a satisfactory answer to a complaint. The Ombudsman can consider complaints from a patient; a close member of the family, partner or representative, if the patient is unable to act for themselves; or from someone who has suffered injustice or hardship as a result of the actions of the NHS. A complaint will normally only be considered within a year of the events which gave rise to it.

The Ombudsman publishes detailed reports of investigations, which identify common themes in complaints. The reports are intended to be used as training tools to improve services, and chief executives are asked to ensure all clinical directors, convenors and complaints managers are aware of them. They are also considered by the House of Commons public administration committee.

www.ombudsman.org.uk

6 Financing the NHS

Sources of funding

Taxation

Funding healthcare through taxation ensures universal access to services irrespective of ability to pay. In 2003/04 more than 90 per cent of NHS funding in England came from general taxation and national insurance contributions: almost three-quarters from general taxation – the Consolidated Fund – and about a fifth from the NHS element of national insurance.

NHS sources of finance 2003–04

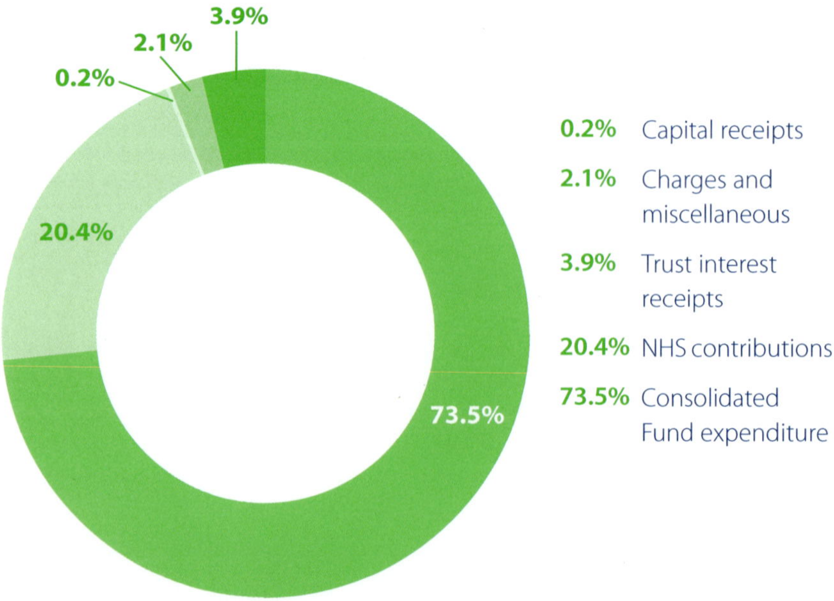

Apart from social security payments, the health service is the biggest single item of public expenditure, absorbing 15 per cent of tax and NICs.

General taxation is generally regarded as being a highly efficient way of financing healthcare: it means the Government has both a strong incentive and the capacity to control costs; administrative costs especially tend to be low. As taxation draws revenue from a wide base, it helps minimise distortions in particular sectors of the economy. The social insurance element of NHS financing in the form of NICs paid by employees and employers, although relatively small, has been found to be highly progressive – that is, what people pay directly reflects what they can afford.

However, financing healthcare through taxation means the overall level of resources is constrained by what the Government judges the economy can afford and what is electorally viable, and choices between what services are and are not provided are made centrally. Many would argue that in the past the UK system has gone too far in controlling expenditure, leading to under-investment in the NHS compared with other countries over many years. The degree of individual choice available to patients has tended to be relatively limited.

Charges

The NHS currently charges for a limited number of clinical services – mainly prescriptions, dental treatments, sight tests, glasses and contact lenses. These out-of-pocket payments account for about 2 per cent of NHS funding. The principle remains that they should be paid only by those who can afford them, with a safety net built into the system so that those who cannot afford to pay do not have to and are not discouraged from seeking advice and treatment. A wide range of exemptions applies, including in most cases young and elderly people and those who are unemployed or on low incomes.

Prescriptions, dental treatment, sight tests

Since April 2004, prescription charges have been £6.40 per item. It is estimated that about 50 per cent of the population of England does not have to pay prescription charges. In 2000, 85 per cent of prescription items dispensed by community pharmacists and appliance contractors in England were free to patients.

Standard dental examination charges are £5.48–£16.84, depending on the length and depth of the examination. Dental patients have to pay 80 per cent of the cost of treatment up to a maximum of £378.

A sight test costs £16.72.

In addition, there are currently limited charges for non-clinical services such as single maternity rooms and car parking.

Road traffic accidents

Since the 1930s hospitals have been entitled by law to collect money for treating road traffic accident victims. A revised, centralised system for this was introduced in 1999, with the aim of streamlining collection of charges from drivers' insurance companies and setting a national tariff of charges to reflect the real costs of treatment.

NHS charges are levied when someone is involved in a road accident, receives examination or treatment at an NHS hospital and subsequently is paid compensation for their injuries. The charges are paid by whoever pays the compensation, and raise about £8 million per month for the NHS in England. The Compensation Recovery Unit, part of the Benefits Agency, collects the charges, which are:

- flat rate for treatment without admission: £452
- daily rate for treatment with admission: £556
- maximum in any one case: £33,000.

Overseas visitors

The Government has announced changes to the legislation that allows the NHS to charge overseas visitors for treatment, extending the scope for charging. The changes are:

- the spouse and dependent children of an overseas visitor resident in the UK will no longer be eligible for free treatment unless they are living with them permanently in the UK
- the rule allowing anyone living in the UK for more than 12 months to be allowed free treatment will no longer apply to those with no legal right to be in the country
- the 12-month residency rule will no longer apply to anyone who comes to the UK specifically for private medical treatment but then remains for more than a year
- those coming to the UK to work will no longer be eligible for free treatment unless their employment is based in the UK
- overseas students here to study full-time will now be fully exempt from charges
- British state pensioners who choose to split their time between the UK and another European Economic Area member state will be exempt from charges for treatment.

Asylum seekers whose application for refuge in the UK is outstanding are entitled to use NHS services without charge.

Other sources
Other sources of NHS funding come from land sales and income generation schemes. In addition, the New Opportunities Fund – which is financed through the National Lottery – provides complementary funding for health (as well as education and the environment). Since 1999 the NOF has funded the Healthy Living Centres initiative (£232 million in England), palliative care for adults with cancer (£23 million), diagnostic equipment to detect cancer (£93 million) and resources for fighting cancer, coronary heart disease and stroke (£232 million).

Further information
New Opportunities Fund: www.nof.org.uk

Resource allocation

The Treasury is responsible for overall public expenditure. Every two years it conducts a comprehensive spending review of all Government departments covering three years. After each review, the Department of Health – like all Government departments – draws up a public service agreement with the Treasury, setting out what it is expected to provide with its new resources over a three-year period. The DoH in turn issues priorities and planning guidance to the NHS.

Spending on the NHS divides into these main programmes:
- *Hospital and community health services,* and discretionary family health services. This covers hospital and community health services, prescribing costs for drugs and appliances and discretionary general medical services (which include reimbursements of GMS GPs' practice staff, premises, out-of-hours and IT expenses). It also includes other centrally funded initiatives, services and special allocations managed centrally by the DoH (such as education and training, and research and development).
- *Family health services non-discretionary.* This covers demand-led family health services, including the remuneration of GPs for items such as capitation payments, health promotion and basic practice allowance, the cost of general dental and ophthalmic services, dispensing remuneration and income from dental and prescription charges.
- *Central health and miscellaneous services,* for example, certain public health functions and support to the voluntary sector.
- *Administration of the Department of Health.*

Role of PCTs

Since 2003/04 the DoH has made allocations covering a three-year period direct to primary care trusts, which now control 81 per cent of the NHS budget. They have to plan the use of their resources over the three years as agreed with their strategic health authority. However, they must manage within their annual resource limit total for each year, although they can carry forward planned underspends of up to 0.25 per cent.

These unified budget allocations cover:

- commissioning hospital, mental health and learning disability services
- providing community services
- PCT running costs
- GP and community nurses' prescribing costs
- primary care infrastructure.

Provided they are achieving the targets in their local delivery plan (see pages 50 – 51) and keep sufficient in reserve to pay GPs, PCTs can use their resources as they see fit.

To commission services for their local populations, PCTs draw up service agreements with healthcare providers – mostly NHS trusts. These agreements typically run for three to five years, and cover cost, volume, quality, efficiency and effectiveness of services.

NHS trusts derive most of their income by providing services in this way, although they also earn some by providing private healthcare and are funded separately for training health professionals. They may also generate some income from shops or car parks on hospital premises.

NHS trusts and PCTs have to publish their costs for individual procedures on a consistent basis in the national schedule of reference costs. This gives details of the unit costs for a range of procedures and treatments, from x-rays to lung transplant surgery and from a visit by a district nurse to a home delivery by a midwife. Commissioners can use the information when negotiating agreements, and identify areas for improving efficiency.

Weighted capitation formula

A weighted capitation formula is used to determine each PCT's target share of resources. This reflects the age distribution of a PCT's population and the health needs it may have due to deprivation or high mortality and morbidity levels, as well as unavoidable geographical variations in the cost of providing services. The intention is that every PCT should be able to commission similar levels of health services for populations in similar need. A wide-ranging review of the formula to make it fairer was recently conducted by the Advisory Committee on Resource Allocation, whose members included NHS managers, GPs and academics. A key criterion of the new formula is the reduction of health inequalities.

The formula takes into account:

- hospital and community health services
- HIV/AIDS
- GP practice infrastructure, such as practice staff wages, premises and equipment
- GP prescribing (drug costs of prescriptions dispensed, not dispensing fees)
- GP remuneration.

These components are used to adjust each PCT's 'crude population' based on 2001 census estimates. Some PCTs will currently be funded above their target level and others below it (this is known as their distance from target), reflecting the legacy of previous years' allocations. Ministers decide for each allocation round the level of increase which all PCTs receive to deliver on national and local priorities and the level of extra resources to PCTs that are under target, to move them closer to their weighted capitation targets.

Further information

Resource allocation: weighted capitation formula, DoH, March 2003.

Spotlight on policy: payment by results

Far-reaching changes are being implemented to the way money flows through the NHS in England between commissioners and providers. A system of payment by results is being introduced in an attempt to ensure funding follows the patient. This is designed to underpin Government policy on increasing patient choice and encouraging a diversity of providers. The changes are being implemented gradually over five years to 2008 in order to monitor the effect and reduce the risks of financial destabilisation.

Spotlight on policy: payment by results – *continued*

The aim is to provide a transparent system for paying trusts which will encourage activity to reduce waiting times. PCTs will commission the volume of activity they require for their populations, but instead of drawing up block agreements with NHS trusts as previously, the trusts and other providers will be paid for the activity they undertake. They will lose money on a cost-per-case basis for failing to deliver the volumes commissioned, and will earn extra on a cost-per-case basis for treating additional patients.

A tariff derived from national reference costs will remove prices from local negotiation, so that commissioners focus instead on gains in patient choice, quality, shorter waiting time, volumes of activity and efficiency. Initially the tariff was applied to 15 healthcare resource groups (HRGs) for elective procedures in ophthalmology, cardiothoracic surgery, ENT, trauma and orthopaedics, general surgery and urology.

HRGs classify patients into clinically similar groups requiring similar levels of resources for diagnosis, treatment and care. The NHS Information Authority has developed HRGs with help from clinicians to reflect clinical practice and patterns of delivery.

Another 33 HRGs are being added in 2004/05, and from then to 2008 the system will extend to cover most significant inpatient, day-case and outpatient activity.

Reforming financial flows in this way is one of the most significant changes in the way the NHS operates. Trusts whose costs exceed the tariff price will face a challenge if they are to avoid deficits. The quality of the data used to construct the reference costs on which the tariff prices are based will be paramount.

Further information

Reforming NHS financial flows: introducing payment by results, DoH, October 2002.
Payment by results: preparing for 2005, DoH, August 2003.

Capital

Allocating capital

Capital allocations are made under three classifications:

- operational capital (formerly known as block capital)
- strategic capital (formerly discretionary capital)
- the access fund.

Operational capital is allocated directly to NHS trusts and PCTs according to a national needs-based formula. It is used to fund smaller developments and to replace or maintain equipment; trusts and PCTs can spend their operational capital as they choose. In 2003/04 operational capital was increased by 10 per cent on the previous year.

Strategic capital is allocated to strategic health authorities according to weighted capitation to fund schemes they decide are priorities for bringing about major change.

The access fund is also allocated to SHAs for them to use as incentives for trusts and PCTs to improve performance. Trusts and PCTs must achieve significant, pre-agreed improvements in access to qualify. A condition of the access fund is that at least 50 per cent of any money awarded must be spent on schemes put forward by the clinical teams that achieved the performance improvement.

In 2003/04, capital allocations were:

- operational capital: £884 million
- strategic capital: £684 million
- access fund: £100 million.

All major investment schemes are submitted to the DoH's capital prioritisation advisory group to be assessed and prioritised according to where health need is greatest. Since it began in 1997, 68 major hospital developments worth over £8.8 billion have been given the go-ahead, 64 under the private finance initiative (PFI, see pages 84–5) and four using public capital.

Spending and borrowing capital

Each tier of the NHS is restricted in the amount of capital it can invest without seeking authorisation.

- The DoH can approve full business cases for public capital financed builds, PFI and IT schemes up to £100 million; Treasury approval is required for cases over £100 million.

- SHAs may approve all trust and PCT business cases up to £25 million. This limit applies to all build, PFI and IT contracts and all investments financed through lease transactions. SHAs have a delegated limit of £5 million for their own business cases of any kind.
- Three-star and two-star trusts' delegated limits are up to £10 million and £8 million respectively depending on their turnover, and apply to build, PFI, IT and equipment investments, although lower limits apply for property leases.
- The basic trust limit for build schemes, IT, equipment investments and property leases is £1 million for one-star and zero-star trusts, regardless of turnover.

The DoH also sets a maximum amount that trusts can borrow. This external financing limit (EFL) is based on the trust's business plan and can be positive, zero or negative. A positive EFL enables a trust to spend capital in excess of its income; a negative EFL means a trust's capital is less than its income, and it must repay the surplus to the Treasury or invest it for future schemes.

A limit is also set on capital-to-revenue transfers to control the amount of capital that can be transferred to support revenue spending.

Priorities for capital investment

Capital investment priorities for 2003/04 included:

- diagnosis and treatment centres (£184 million)
- cancer (£100 million)
- coronary heart disease (£103 million)
- mental health (£29 million)
- primary care (£120 million)
- information management and technology (£370 million)
- improving disinfection facilities (£40 million).

The total capital budget in 2003/04 was just over £4 billion, including £227 million from land sales and £901 million from the private finance initiative.

Private finance initiative (PFI)

PFI involves a public-private partnership between an NHS organisation and a private sector consortium that makes private capital available for health service projects. All major NHS capital projects are expected to consider whether PFI could represent a value-for-money solution.

The private sector consortium will usually include a construction company, a funding organisation and a facilities management provider. Contracts for major PFI schemes may be for 30 years or more and are typically DBFO (design, build, finance and operate), which means the private sector partner is responsible for:

- designing the facilities (based on the requirements specified by the NHS)
- building the facilities (to time and at a fixed cost)
- financing the capital cost (with the return to be recovered through continuing to make the facilities available and meeting the NHS's requirements)
- operating the facilities (providing facilities management and other support services).

PFI schemes must demonstrate value for money, which is usually achieved by the PFI partner assuming risks which would otherwise have been borne by the public sector, and by efficiency savings. The PFI contract sets out the performance standards required of the consortium. The NHS makes no payments until services are provided to the agreed standard, and then they must be maintained to ensure full payment.

The aims of PFI are to reduce the overall risks associated with procuring new assets and services for the NHS, and to improve the quality and cost-effectiveness of public services. Because the PFI partner's capital is at risk, they have an incentive to perform well throughout the life of the contract, while private sector management, commercial and creative skills are harnessed for the NHS's benefit.

Critics have questioned whether PFI will really provide long-term value for money for the NHS, and have claimed services have been cut in some cases to make schemes affordable. In response the Government has said: 'PFI is only a procurement tool – not an end in itself – and will only be used in cases where it offers value for money to the taxpayer and the NHS.' It is not advised in projects involving rapid change, such as IT.

Currently 114 hospital schemes are in progress – 104 under PFI and ten financed with public capital. Of the 100 hospital schemes announced in the NHS Plan, 31 are already operational, and 27 of them were delivered under PFI. In addition, 40 medium-sized PFI schemes, including mental health and community services, have been approved, of which 11 are already operational.

NHS Local Improvement Finance Trust (LIFT)

NHS LIFT aims to encourage investment in primary care and community-based facilities and services to achieve the NHS Plan target of 500 one-stop primary care centres and the refurbishment or replacement of up to 3,000 GP premises. It is similar to PFI, except that public capital is involved and stakeholders include PCTs, local authorities and GPs.

Partnerships for Health, a public–private partnership between the DoH and Partnerships UK, is investing money in NHS LIFT and helping to attract additional private funding. There are currently 42 LIFT schemes in England, many in deprived inner cities. NHS LIFT seeks investment in primary care developments by bundling them together. Local LIFT schemes rent accommodation to GPs, pharmacists, opticians, dentists and others on a lease basis. An initial £200 million of public money was used to kick-start LIFT, which has attracted investment so far of about £1 billion.

NHS spending

Budget 2002

From the time the NHS was founded until the end of the 1990s, its annual average increase in funding was just over 3 per cent – slightly more than the real growth in the economy as a whole. However, from the early 1980s, real spending changes were erratic. Taking into account the level of inflation in the NHS rather than in the general economy, annual average growth was about 0.9 per cent from 1983 to 1987, 2 per cent from 1987 to 1992 and 1.4 per cent from 1992 to 1997.

In 2000 the Government announced its intention to raise health spending to the EU average, and in 2001 Derek Wanless was commissioned to produce the first evidence-based assessment of the NHS's long-term resource requirements (see pages 89–90).

As a result, the Chancellor announced in his 2002 Budget major increases in NHS spending until 2007/08: it is set to rise from £53.5 billion to £87.1 billion. These are the largest sustained increases in any five-year period in NHS history: an annual average increase of 7.4 per cent in real terms between 2002/03 and 2007/08, a total increase of 43 per cent in real terms over the period. This translates into a rise in NHS cash spending per household from £2,370 in 2001/02 to £4,060 in 2007/08. The aim is to put the NHS on a 'sound long-term financial footing', making significant investment in IT, buildings and equipment. To help pay for these increases, national insurance contributions were raised by 1 per cent from April 2003.

Efficiency savings

Spending increases usually come with caveats about the level of efficiency savings the NHS is expected to make. The current priorities and planning guidance states:

> Reports to stakeholders will need to show how extra funding has been used, in every case demonstrating that the organisation has added value to at least the level of the funding and secured a minimum 1 per cent cost-efficiency increase as well as an increase in quality equivalent to 1 per cent of its budget.

Key organisation: NHS Bank

The NHS Bank provides grants or loans to organisations with financial problems that threaten to have an unacceptable impact on patient services. It is intended to operate at arm's length from the DoH, replacing a system of brokerage in which NHS trusts with a cash surplus were able to lend to others. It was set up in 2002 with £100 million and is managed by four strategic health authority chief executives with the DoH's finance director as chair. The full £100 million was allocated to three SHAs that year. A further £100 million was made available for the subsequent three years. SHAs applying for assistance need to produce performance improvement plans with proposals to restore financial stability, timescales for achieving it and their underlying assumptions.

Where the money is spent

NHS total net expenditure (revenue and capital) in England in 2003/04 was expected to be over £63 billion. The largest part of NHS spending is on hospital and community health services, discretionary family health services and related services. For 2003/04, planned net revenue expenditure is £53.7 billion and planned net capital expenditure is £2.9 billion. Within overall NHS net expenditure, the total for non-discretionary family health services is expected to account for £5.5 billion. The remainder will be spent on central health and miscellaneous services.

NHS planned net expenditure 2003–04

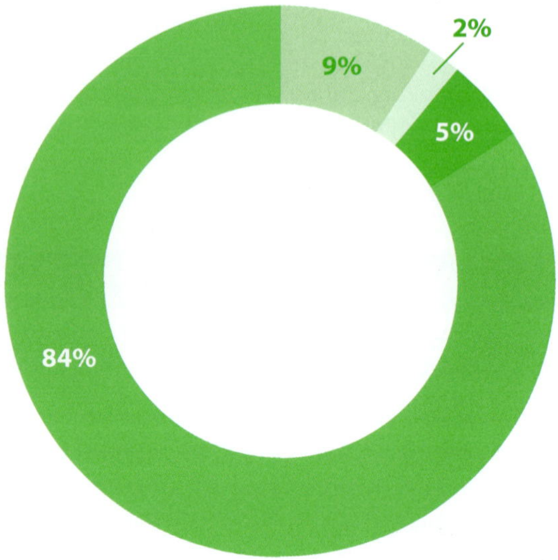

84% HCFHS

9% FHS non-discretionary

5% HCHS capital

2% CHMS

Total £63,294 million

Hospital and community health services gross current expenditure by sector, 2000–01

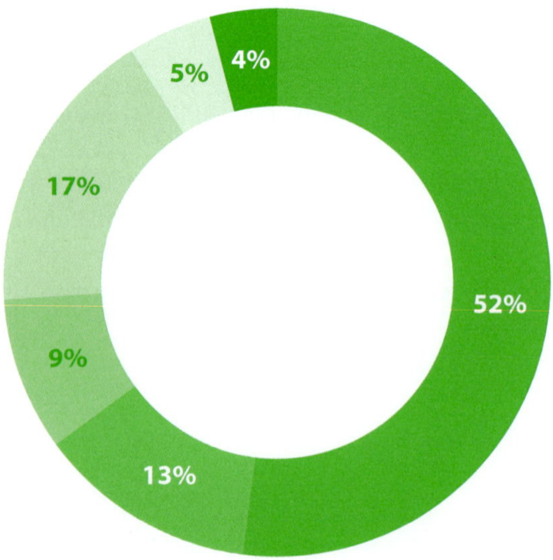

4% Maternity £1,205m

5% Learning disability £1,486m

9% Elderly £2,640m

13% Mental Health £3,826m

17% Other £5,351m

52% Acute £15,500m

Total £30,008 million

Within spending on hospital and community health services, acute services dominate. This reflects the demand for emergency treatment, and the continuing emphasis on reducing waiting lists and waiting times. About 12 per cent is spent on mental health services, 10 per cent on services for elderly people, 5 per cent on people with learning disabilities and 5 per cent on maternity services. Healthcare for people over 65 accounts for around 40 per cent of the total expenditure.

European comparisons

In 1997 the UK's public and private health spending as a proportion of national income (gross domestic product or GDP) ranked 14th out of the 15 European Union countries, while its public sector health spending was 11th. In 2000 the Prime Minister pledged to raise NHS spending as a proportion of GDP so that it would equal the European average – then about 8 per cent – within five years. There is some debate about how best to calculate the EU average, but broadly the increases announced in the 2002 Budget look set to achieve this aim, raising NHS spending to a projected 9.4 per cent of GDP by 2007/08.

Measuring inflation

Increases in the cost of goods and services used by the NHS are measured by the health service cost index (HSCI). The HSCI weights together price increases for a broad range of items – for example drugs, medical equipment, fuel and telephone charges. Calculations are based on spending on these items reported in financial returns. Between 1992 and 2000, net NHS expenditure increased by 43 per cent in cash terms, by 17.4 per cent when inflation in the economy as a whole was taken into account and by 14.1 per cent after accounting for NHS-specific inflation.

Key text: Wanless Report

In 2001 the Chancellor commissioned Derek Wanless, former chief executive of the NatWest Bank, to examine demand and cost pressures in the NHS over the next 20 years and recommend the spending needed for a 'publicly funded, comprehensive, high-quality service available on the basis of clinical need and not ability to pay'. The Wanless review team published an interim report for consultation in November 2001 and its final report in April 2002.

Wanless found that although an ageing population would be an important influence, this would not be the main factor driving up costs. Patients were likely to demand more choice and higher-quality services. Improving information and communication technology would be key to achieving this, while the NHS would have to change its skill-mix and ways of working, and enhance the role of primary care.

Key text: Wanless Report – *continued*

Wanless concluded that spending would need to rise between 9.4 per cent and 11.3 per cent of GDP in 20 years' time, with the fastest growth before 2008. He warned: 'Both additional resources and radical reform are vital: neither would succeed without the other.'

Wanless's figures assume that plans for huge expansion of the workforce are achieved, that IT spend can be doubled and used productively while the NHS fulfils commitments on waiting times and national service frameworks. If productivity improvement falls short of 2 per cent a year, spending will need to rise to an even higher proportion of GDP.

His review endorsed decentralising the NHS, and argued that targets 'should be used with care'. There should be stability and certainty of funding, taking account of local needs without creating perverse incentives. He called too for greater transparency and better understanding of healthcare costs.

Securing our future: taking a long-term view. Final report, HM Treasury, April 2002. www.hm-treasury.gov.uk

Shared financial services

The shared financial services initiative has been developed to improve the quality and value for money of NHS financial services by sharing knowledge, skills and resources. Currently two shared service centres (SSCs) exist, with 26 trusts taking part in the pilot in West Yorkshire and 15 in the south-west, transferring some of their financial processes to the two centres. The centres – in Leeds and Bristol – work as one organisation on two sites.

They are purpose-designed for processing financial business support information. Dealing with orders and invoices and paying suppliers are split between the two SSCs. West Yorkshire scans invoices into the system on behalf of all the pilot trusts, and South West produces all output documents – for example, purchase orders and cheques for the customer organisations. Staff involved in any finance function, from budget-holding to petty cash, will use the new shared financial services system.

The SSCs have been made possible by the advent of online electronic systems accessed via the internet. This allows processing of business transactions from anywhere in the country via a telecommunications link.

As Government policy is to devolve more responsibility to NHS organisations, it is not mandatory to make use of shared financial services. The SSCs' future may therefore lie in a joint venture with private sector partners or as a non-departmental public body.

Further information

www.sharedfinancialservices.co.uk

Buying goods and services

Pharmaceutical Price Regulation Scheme

The PPRS regulates the prices of branded medicines and the profits that manufacturers are allowed to make on their sales to the NHS. It is a voluntary agreement made between the DoH and the Association of the British Pharmaceutical Industry. A series of voluntary agreements has limited branded medicine prices and profits since 1957, each lasting five years or so.

Agreements cover all licensed, branded prescription medicines sold to the NHS. They do not cover products without a brand name (generics) nor over-the-counter branded products except when prescribed by a doctor. The PPRS is a UK-wide scheme and covers around 80 per cent by value of the medicines used in the NHS in both primary and secondary care, worth about £7 billion.

The PPRS seeks to achieve reasonable prices for the NHS, while recognising that the industry needs to earn the money to enable it to develop and market new and improved medicines. The agreement ending in September 2004 secured a 4.5 per cent price reduction for the NHS which delivered annual savings of £250 million. It requires companies to seek the DoH's agreement for price increases. Those with NHS sales of more than £25 million a year must submit annual data on sales, costs, assets and profitability and repay the excess where profits exceed the agreed return on capital.

A maximum price scheme for generics – on which the NHS spends £1 billion a year – was introduced in 2000 to restrain the drugs bill after steep price rises, saving around £330 million a year. From 2004 a new scheme has come into force under which, where there is a limited number of manufacturers of a generic medicine or the supply is concentrated, manufacturers have to seek the DoH's agreement to any price increase. Manufacturers and wholesalers must submit quarterly information for income revenues, cost of purchases and volumes of transactions.

NHS Purchasing and Supply Agency

This agency is responsible for ensuring the NHS gets the best value for money when purchasing other goods and services. It acts as a centre of expertise and knowledge in purchasing and supply matters, and contracts on a national basis for products and services which are strategically critical to the NHS. It also acts where large-scale purchasing power will yield greater savings than those achieved by contracting on a local or regional basis.

PASA works with 400 NHS organisations and manages 3,000 national purchasing contracts, influencing around half the £7 billion the NHS spends on goods and services.

Further information

www.pasa.doh.gov.uk

Key organisation: NHS Counter Fraud and Security Management Service

CFSMS is a special health authority set up in 2003 to prevent, detect and investigate fraud and corruption, and manage security in the NHS. It aims to 'create an anti-fraud culture, maximise deterrence of fraud, successfully prevent fraud which cannot be deterred and promptly detect fraud which cannot be prevented'. It hopes to permanently reduce fraud to a minimum, releasing resources for patient services. Its security management arm is particularly concerned with staff and patient safety, maternity unit security and the security of medicines and hazardous materials. Its predecessor body, the NHS Counter Fraud Service, reduced pharmaceutical and dental patient fraud by 41 per cent and 25 per cent respectively, and cut optical patient fraud from £13 million to £10 million.

www.cfsms.nhs.uk.

7 Human resources

The NHS Plan declared:

> NHS staff are a precious resource. They are what make the NHS tick. A modern NHS must offer staff a better deal in their working lives. It is never an easy life working in the NHS but it can be a better life.

As the UK's largest employer – indeed, one of the largest employers in the world – the NHS must attach special importance to good human resources policy and practice. Staff costs account for about 75 per cent of its expenditure. Current priorities for the health service include expanding staff numbers and becoming a model employer. Effective recruitment, retention and remuneration of a well-trained and well-motivated workforce are seen as crucial factors in achieving the Government's ambitions for patient care.

Staff numbers

Approximately 1.3 million people were employed by more than 600 NHS organisations in England in September 2003 (the latest figures available) on a headcount basis. This represents an increase of 60,000 since 2002 and an average increase of 37,000 a year since 1997.

The NHS Plan pledged a major and rapid expansion in NHS staff numbers. Targets in the priorities and planning framework 2003–06 are that by 2004, compared with 1999, there would be:

- 7,500 more consultants
- 2,000 more GPs
- 1,000 more specialist registrars
- 550 more GP registrars
- 20,000 more nurses
- over 6,500 more therapists and other health professionals.

At September 2003, progress was as follows:

- 5,429 more consultants (72 per cent of target)
- 1,891 more GPs (95 per cent of target)
- 1,937 more specialist registrars (target achieved)
- 715 more GP registrars (target achieved)
- 56,722 more nurses (target achieved)
- 8,026 more therapists and other health professionals (target achieved).

In total, there were:

- 108,993 doctors
- 386,359 qualified nurses, midwives, health visitors and practice nurses
- 122,066 qualified scientific, therapeutic and technical staff
- 15,957 qualified ambulance staff
- 298,752 support staff to doctors and nurses
- 52,230 scientific, therapeutic and technical support staff
- 9,684 ambulance support staff
- 92,257 NHS infrastructure support staff in central functions
- 72,230 staff in hotel, property and estates
- 35,321 managers and senior managers
- 88,424 GP practice staff, excluding practice nurses.

The NHS has therefore made good progress on tackling workforce shortages, but more needs to be done to maintain the momentum and increase the numbers of medical staff. This is particularly important as the NHS will face a retirement bulge in the next few years when increasing numbers of healthcare workers reach retirement age and competition with other employers to recruit staff remains keen.

Further information

HR in the NHS Plan, DoH, July 2002.
Delivering the HR in the NHS Plan 2003, DoH, June 2003.

Management numbers: myth and reality

As the NHS expands capacity, it is employing more managers and support staff, as well as more doctors and nurses. While the growth in medical and nursing staff has met universal approval, the expansion in support workers has excited hostile comment and suspicion that the service is squandering its extra resources on bureaucracy.

Yet the service could no more function without them than it could without doctors and nurses: indeed, many have a clinical background and they perform a wide variety of tasks, often involving direct patient contact. Support staff undoubtedly form a large part of the NHS workforce:

clinical support staff: 28 per cent
of which:
- 42 per cent are nursing assistants or auxiliaries

infrastructure support staff: 15 per cent
of which:
- 13 per cent are managers
- 7 per cent are senior managers
- 47 per cent work in finance, HR and IT
- 33 per cent work in hotel, property and estates, including cleaners laundry catering and maintenance staff.

As a proportion of all NHS staff, managers (23,265) account for 1.8 per cent and senior managers (12,056) for 0.9 per cent. To put these figures in perspective, there are:
- 11 qualified nurses for every manager
- three doctors for every manager
- 2.4 hospital consultants for every senior manager.

Growth in support staff has been in direct response to policy initiatives to improve the quality of care. These command broad support, yet their administrative ramifications are easily overlooked. For example, many of the new posts are for bed managers and discharge co-ordinators, or for receptionists, telephonists and switchboard operators – whose numbers some trusts may seek to boost to provide a more efficient response to patients and the public. Offering patients a specific time and date in advance for their appointments rather than expecting them to arrive in blocks throughout the day is now regarded as best practice, and has complicated the booking clerk's role. Telephoning patients to remind them of appointments reduces 'did not attends', but is one among an array of additional duties that could lead a trust to reinforce its clerical workforce.

Key organisation: NHS Professionals

NHS Professionals is a special health authority (see page 14) which acts as an in-house agency for supplying temporary staff. It was established in 2000 to match healthcare staff seeking temporary work with the NHS trusts who need them, so that they do not have to rely exclusively on commercial recruitment firms. NHS Professionals is responsible for strategic oversight of temporary labour markets and management of agency framework contracts, setting standards and policy for NHS temporary staffing. It currently has more than 40,000 on its books, and aims to cover all trusts by 2005.

www.nhsprofessionals.nhs.uk

The importance of good HR in health services

Common sense suggests that an organisation will run more effectively if its staff are treated well and are happy in their work. Recent academic research has found evidence to back bold assertions about the relationship between good HR practice and better patient outcomes.

Work by Aston Business School has established that hospitals with progressive people management policies achieve better patient outcomes, including lower mortality rates. Researchers examined HR practices in 61 NHS acute hospitals in England across all occupational groups, and also looked at deaths following emergency surgery or hip fracture and overall mortality rates. Data from primary care had already shown that innovation was much greater where team working was good; people in well functioning teams also tended to suffer less stress. The study was controlled for factors such as the number of doctors per bed, local health needs and hospital size.

They found that 33 per cent of the variation in the hospitals' standardised mortality ratios could be explained by knowledge of their HR practices. Appraisals had the strongest association with lower mortality rates: improving the extent and sophistication of a hospital's appraisal system would lead to a 12.3 per cent drop in deaths after hip fractures. Increasing the number of existing staff working in teams would result in 7.1 per cent fewer deaths. Where the trust's HR director was a voting member of the board, the relationship between progressive people management practices and patient outcomes was even stronger – suggesting the importance of HR directors having appropriate powers to bring about change.

Further information

Action Point 33: Good HR, better patient care, NHS Confederation, August 2002.
www.abs.aston.ac.uk

The four pillars

According to the strategy set out in HR in the NHS Plan, good HR practice in the NHS rests on four pillars.

Pillar 1: making the NHS a model employer

Making the NHS a model employer will help attract new recruits and improve the working lives of existing staff. The Government wants the NHS to be seen as 'the' place to work – the employer of choice. For this, it needs to offer good working conditions, the ability to balance life in and outside work, job security, lifelong learning and fair pay. Staff also need to feel involved in decision making. Good leadership, teamworking and effective communication are also key. To this end, NHS organisations are being encouraged to sign up to the Improving Working Lives standard, which commits them to creating well-managed, flexible working environments which support staff, promote their welfare and development, and respect the need for a balance between work and their home life. Over 90 per cent of organisations that should have achieved accreditation had done so by April 2003, as had most PCTs.

Other measures include the NHS childcare strategy, which has set a target of providing 150 extra on-site nurseries and access for all staff to a childcare co-ordinator; 120 new nursery schemes have been opened or are in the pipeline and 155 childcare co-ordinators are in post so far. A flexible careers scheme now allows doctors to take a break from full-time work while retaining their clinical skills. New initiatives to protect the health of staff have seen some trusts significantly reduce sickness rates.

Pillar 2: ensuring the NHS provides a model career

Staff should have opportunities to develop and extend their careers through lifelong learning so they can move up the 'skills escalator'. At the same time, roles and workload can be passed down the escalator if appropriate. Employers benefit from a structured programme of skills development that supports recruitment and retention of staff, developing them to fill posts traditionally hard to fill.

A network of more than 30 external partner organisations has been set up to help disseminate the skills escalator concept. Modernising pay (see page 103), setting up the NHSU to promote learning and personal development (see opposite), reforming professional regulation (see page 67) and workforce development (see pages 68-70) are all intended to enhance the attractiveness of a career in the health service.

Pillar 3: improving staff morale

Morale, motivation and job satisfaction improve if staff feel they work for a respected, high-profile and effective organisation. Good communications can have a significant impact on morale – as can negative publicity about the NHS. The zero-tolerance policy on violence in the workplace is an important initiative here, as is the national staff opinion survey carried out by the Healthcare Commission in 2003.

Pillar 4: building people management skills

High-quality patient care needs effective organisations with strong leadership, clear strategies and business plans with explicit criteria to monitor performance, as the Aston research has shown (see page 96).

Training

Increasing the numbers of staff in training is vital to increasing and sustaining the size of the NHS workforce. The NHS Plan pledged that by 2004 there would be:

- 5,500 more nurses, midwives and health visitors being trained each year
- 4,450 more therapists and other key professional staff being trained
- 1,000 more specialist registrars – the key feeder grade for consultants – targeting key specialities
- 450 more doctors training for general practice.

Four new medical schools and three centres of medical education opened in 2003, increasing the number of medical school places by over 2,000, the largest increase in medical school places since 1948. Progress on other targets by 2002 was:

- 3,063 more training places for nurses and midwives (56 per cent of target)
- 1,838 more training places for therapists and other key professionals (41 per cent of target).

Key organisation: NHSU

NHSU is still at an early stage of development, but is the NHS's corporate 'university' for health and social care staff at all levels and has pledged to 'create a culture that makes learning a central part of everyone's working life'. It also plans to provide learning opportunities for patients, carers and the public.

Programmes so far include an induction course designed for everyone who joins the NHS, a masters-level programme which will equip nurses, allied health professionals and paramedics to see, treat and refer patients, and a job guarantee scheme which helps longer-term unemployed people into health and social care careers. Other programmes and services will be rolled out during 2004 and beyond.

NHSU has a major role in providing access to mentoring, library and information services, and forming learning communities. Its three core strategies are to:
- create a comprehensive, coherent, high-quality learning environment for health and social care staff
- transform learning opportunities
- lead research into learning needs and outcomes.

It intends to avoid duplicating existing provision or competing with established providers, but as well as developing its own learning programmes, it will act as a broker for existing facilities, resources and provision, adapting them where necessary.

Warwick University will be its principal national academic partner, together with 11 others in the regions, working mainly in consortia.

www.nhsu.nhs.uk

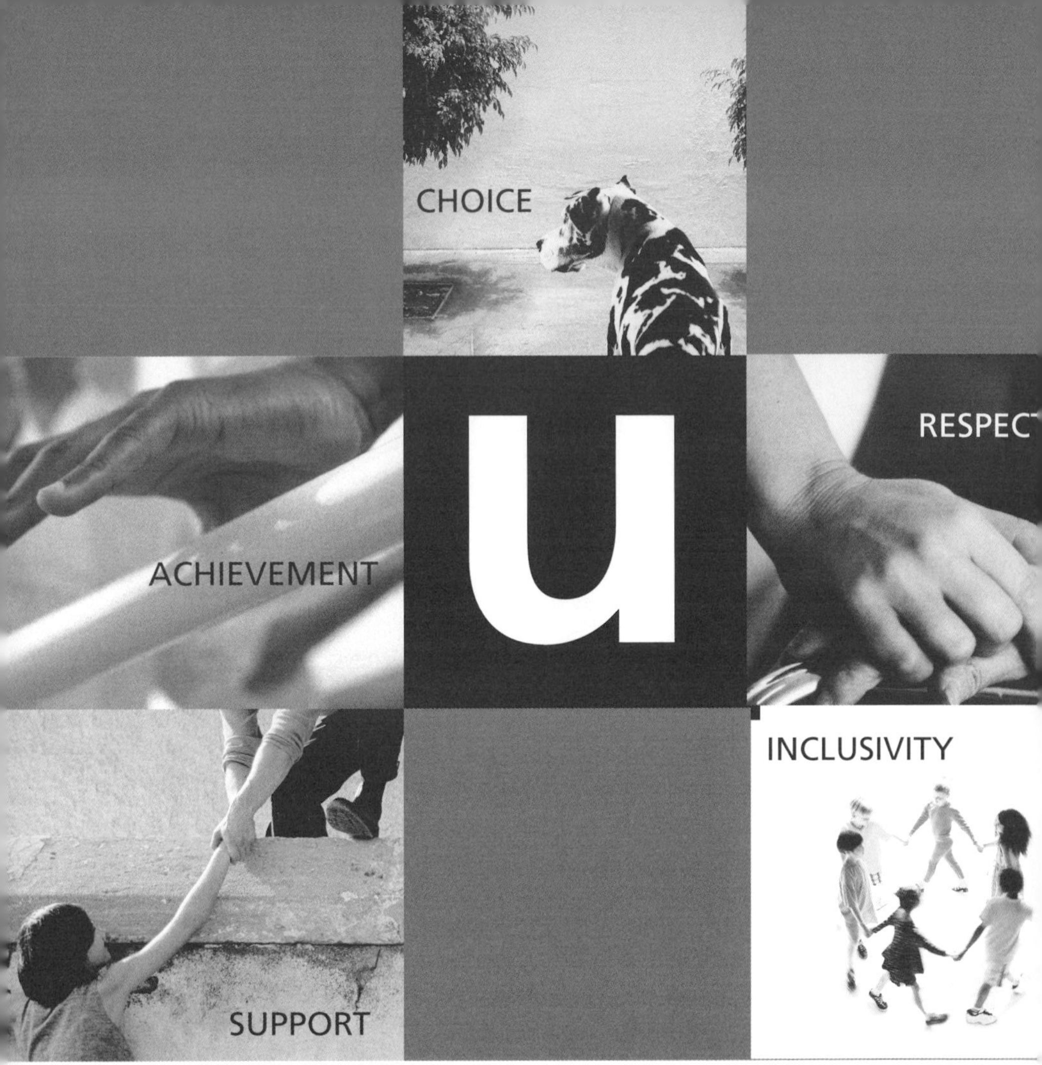
CHOICE
ACHIEVEMENT
u
RESPECT
SUPPORT
INCLUSIVITY

Medical education and the medical Royal Colleges

The Postgraduate Medical Education and Training Board (PMETB), set up in 2003, brings together responsibility for all postgraduate medical education and assesses doctors completing final postgraduate training. It oversees standards relating to medical training in the NHS and elsewhere, acting independently of Government. It has no responsibility for undergraduate medical education, which is overseen by the General Medical Council.

The PMETB comprises 25 members – 16 medical and nine lay (including the chair). Six are taken from a list provided by the Academy of Medical Royal Colleges and one from a list provided by the GMC. Of the 25, the Secretary of State for Health appoints 19 members, and the administrations in Scotland, Wales and Northern Ireland appoint one medical and one lay member each.

The 14 medical Royal Colleges and their faculties remain important elements in medical education and training. Each Royal College aims to ensure high-quality care by improving standards and influencing policy and practice. They conduct membership examinations which are specific to their particular speciality, and which represent the level of clinical ability which doctors must attain to become consultants. The Colleges help define and monitor education and training, support doctors in their practice, and advise the Government, public and the profession on healthcare issues. Their representative body is the Academy of Medical Royal Colleges.

Modernising medical careers

The Government has put forward proposals for restructuring postgraduate medical training. All graduates leaving medical school will enter a two-year foundation programme designed to provide a solid grounding in practical medicine and develop core clinical skills. Doctors will also be required to enhance their communication, team working and IT skills. At the end of the programme they will be ready to enter speciality training and continue their career development.

Further information

www.mmc.nhs.uk/index.asp

Modernising medical careers – the next steps: the future shape of foundation, specialist and general practice training programmes, UK Health Departments, April 2004.

Nursing education

Education for nursing takes place at university at either diploma or degree level, with placements in local hospital and the community. Courses are half theory and half practice. The first year is a common foundation programme, followed by specialisation in adult, children's, mental health or learning disability nursing. Full-time diploma courses last three years; degree courses last three or four years. Midwifery education is also at diploma or degree level.

The nursing cadet scheme, run by NHS trusts in England, enables those without qualifications for university entry to undertake an initial training programme leading to an NVQ level 3 or access-to-nursing qualification. Candidates are then seconded to a university to take a nursing diploma, leading to registration as a nurse.

Management education and training

The NHS general management training scheme (GMTS) is an intensive two-year programme combining early responsibility in real jobs with management education. It includes a ten-week induction and orientation to the NHS, two nine-month work placements, and the opportunity to spend three months working outside the NHS either on secondment to a major company, a posting abroad, project management work in another healthcare organisation or a piece of original research. The scheme has 90 places.

There are also financial management and HR management training schemes with 65 and 12 places respectively. All three schemes are intended for graduates, although applicants to GMTS may be considered if they have a health or management related degree-level equivalent vocational qualification.

Key organisation: NHS Leadership Centre

Part of the NHS Modernisation Agency, the Leadership Centre develops programmes designed for people at all levels in the health service, from frontline staff to those in the most senior roles, clinical and non-clinical. It contributes to policy development on leadership and leadership development, and conducts research into effective leadership. It is also committed to promoting diversity of leadership in the NHS.

www.modern.nhs.uk

Pay

New pay structure

Until recently the NHS's pay structure had undergone little fundamental change, and was seen as arcane and unhelpful. It did not provide equal pay to different staff doing jobs of equal value. For employers it was inflexible and over-complex. It often appeared to get in the way of service improvement and modernisation rather than supporting it.

In 2003 agreement was reached on a new pay structure first proposed in outline in the *Agenda for change* white paper published in 1999 and subsequent related documents. Subject to final agreement from staff organisations, it will apply to all directly employed NHS staff except those covered by the doctors' and dentists' pay review body and senior managers. Staff currently on local contracts will have a choice whether or not to move on to the new system, which is being tested in 12 pilot sites before implementation across the NHS from October 2004.

The new system's guiding principle is that staff who take on new responsibilities get extra rewards. It is based on job evaluation, so that basic pay will reflect knowledge, responsibility, skills and effort, rather than the historic job title or occupational group. To progress fully through the system, staff will need to demonstrate their competence is appropriate to their level of responsibility.

Over the three years to 2005/06 the package in total will be worth on average 12.5 per cent on basic pay. The proposed deal will give a 10 per cent pay increase over three years for all staff, plus an average 5.9 per cent in the longer run.

The new pay system is intended to bring about these changes:

- new working practices will abolish old-fashioned demarcations as the opportunity of extra pay encourages staff to take on new responsibilities
- a more sensible division of labour with nurses, therapists and healthcare assistants taking on new roles that will improve overall NHS productivity, reducing pressures on doctors and other senior clinicians
- clearer rewards for staff who work flexibly outside normal working hours so helping make NHS services more widely available in the evenings and at weekends
- freedom and flexibility for local NHS employers to create new types of jobs and pay staff more in high-cost areas, with London standing to gain most initially from enhanced regional pay
- more staff being recruited and retained as pay, career and training prospects all improve

- a clearer connection between rewards and responsibilities, with pay linked to staff demonstrating their competence, so improving the overall quality of NHS patient care
- abolition of the 1948 pay machinery's 11 different Whitely Councils, 650 different grades, and several thousand different allowances.

New contract for GPs

GPs accepted a new contract for general medical services (GMS) in 2003, which aims to reward practices for higher-quality care, improve GPs' working lives, and ensure patients benefit from a wider range of services in the community.

The key features are:

- The contract is between the primary care trust and the practice rather than with each GP. This is intended to give practices greater freedom to design services for local needs while encouraging better teamworking and skill-mix.
- Help for GPs to manage their workload by enabling practices to transfer some services – including out-of-hours care – to their PCT.
- A quality and outcomes framework which resources and rewards GPs on the basis of how well they care for patients rather than the number they treat. It is hoped this will lead to good chronic disease management in the community to relieve pressures on hospitals.
- A new allocation formula, removing the historic inequality of per-doctor payments which penalise practices in under-doctored areas. Resources will be allocated more fairly, based on patient need, practice workload and costs. A minimum income guarantee will protect practices from losing out under the formula.
- Measures to tackle GP shortages, including a new career structure, protected time for skills development, family-friendly working practices, an enhanced seniority scheme and improved pension arrangements.
- Measures to ensure patients have more choice and access to a wider range of high-quality services, with more treatment in the community rather than the hospital.
- New career opportunities for practice staff, including nurses and practice managers.
- A major overhaul and modernisation of GP premises and their IM&T systems.

Further information

www.nhsconfed.org/gmscontract

New contract for consultants

The new consultants' contract, agreed in 2003, is designed to provide a more effective system of planning and timetabling consultants' duties and activities for the NHS. It will give NHS employers the ability to manage consultants' time in ways that best meet local service needs and priorities. For consultants, it will mean greater transparency about the commitments expected of them and greater clarity over the support they need from employers to make the maximum effective contribution to improving patient services.

Existing consultants must be given the opportunity to take up the new contract and have the choice whether or not to do so, but NHS employers will not offer different types of new contracts in future. Nor will they offer any other contract to newly appointed consultants.

The main features are:

- A new system of mandatory job planning with annual reviews, applying to all consultants. Employers will draw up and agree job plans with the consultant, setting out a consultant's duties, responsibilities and objectives. Job plans will also set out agreed service and related personal objectives.
- A working week for a full-time consultant comprising ten programmed activities of four hours each. This framework will typically allow around three-quarters of a consultant's programmed activities to be devoted to direct clinical care and a quarter to supporting professional activities.
- A 15 per cent average increase in career earnings, taking into account the new salary structure, on-call availability supplements and the likely level of additional programmed activities, and a 24 per cent increase in the maximum basic salary. Progress up the pay scale will not be automatic, but based on consistently meeting job plan requirements, making best endeavours to achieve agreed individual objectives and demonstrating commitment to the NHS.
- All emergency work that takes place at regular and predictable times to be programmed into the working week and counting towards a consultant's programmed activities. Less predictable emergency work should be handled through on-call arrangements. Consultants who need to be on an on-call rota will be paid a supplement on top of their basic salary.
- Non-emergency work outside 7am to 7pm on weekdays and all non-emergency work at weekends to be undertaken only by agreement. There is enhanced recognition for all work outside 7am to 7pm on weekdays, and all work at weekends.
- Consultants to offer the NHS one session of four hours per week before doing private practice.

- A new clinical excellence award scheme to replace the existing distinction award scheme. It will reward consultants who show the greatest commitment to delivering, developing and managing a high-quality service or the greatest levels of achievement in research or teaching. The maximum award under the scheme will be £65,000.
- A new national disciplinary framework to replace the existing local and national procedures.

Further information

NHS Modernisation Agency Consultant Contract Implementation Team (CCIT), www.modern.nhs.uk

A new role for the NHS Confederation in employment issues

The NHS Confederation has built up a considerable record of work on employment issues, as well as being the representative body for NHS organisations. It played a major part in securing the new contract for GPs, acting on the Department of Health's behalf in negotiations, and contributed to the consultants' contract and *Agenda for change.*

It has long influenced HR policy and given evidence on behalf of NHS management to the pay review bodies. The Government has also commissioned the Confederation to undertake other employment-related projects on behalf of the service – such as the review of the NHS pension scheme and the launch of NHS Executive Search, which connects health service organisations with 13 executive search firms, reducing what would otherwise be a lengthy tendering and contracting process.

Now that the Government wants to devolve a far greater range of employment responsibilities, the Confederation will provide an employers' organisation (EO) service.

The EO is intended to be the authoritative voice for the NHS on employment and human resources issues. Its main responsibilities will be to take responsibility for all national pay negotiations, to draw together NHS employers' views on how to implement health service employment policy frameworks and represent them nationally. It will also support implementation of the plans outlined in *Agenda for change* and the new GMS and consultants' contracts.

A new role for the NHS Confederation in employment issues – *continued*

The move is in line with the DoH's policy of devolving responsibility from the centre. About 50 posts will be transferred from the DoH to the EO, covering national pay negotiations, disciplinary frameworks, recruitment campaigns and HR communications.

The EO will be able to represent the interests of local management and the service, enabling trade unions to represent their members' interests and the Government to set the policy objectives and funding framework. This is in keeping with what happens elsewhere in the public sector.

The roles and responsibilities being devolved to the EO include:

- national negotiations, including providing evidence for the pay review bodies
- pursuing national employment issues, such as recruitment, retention and diversity
- research and intelligence – for example, to support work on national negotiations
- guidance and advice for NHS employers, including significant support in cases of a major new contract or legislative change
- communications with stakeholders, including promoting the NHS as an employer.

Performance management and local dispute resolution will not be part of the EO's role. The EO will be an England-only organisation.

It is hoped the benefits for the NHS will be improved HR policy and practice. The EO should be more responsive to employer needs and views, giving them responsibility for the employment agenda. The key challenge for the new EO is expected to be managing relationships with Government and the trade unions as an independent, responsive voice for NHS employers.

www.nhsconfed.org/ourpriorities/employers_organisation.asp

Spotlight on policy: European Working Time Directive

The European Working Time Directive from the Council of the European Union aims to protect the health and safety of EU workers by laying down minimum requirements for working hours, rest periods, annual leave and working arrangements for night workers.

The directive took effect in the UK from 1998 with a few exceptions, including doctors in training. From August 2004 it will be extended to these doctors, too, although it will be phased in with a maximum-hours requirement reducing from 58 hours in 2004 to 48 hours in 2009. GPs are not covered by it as they are self-employed.

The Department of Health says: 'The changes to the NHS when doctors in training come under the remit of the European working-time directive cannot be underestimated. It will be impossible to continue delivering services in the same way that we have done in the past and the staff affected by these changes will include those in many different staff groups.'

The main features are:

- no more than 48 hours work per week
- 11 hours' continuous rest in 24 hours
- 24 hours' continuous rest in seven days (or 48 hours in 14 days)
- 20-minute break in work periods over six hours
- four weeks' annual leave
- for night workers, an average of no more than eight hours' work in 24 over the reference period.

In addition, a case in the European Court of Justice on behalf of a group of Spanish doctors resulted in the SiMAP ruling, which says: 'Time spent on call by doctors … must be regarded in its entirety as working time… if they are required to be present at the health centre.' This means that resident on-call working patterns in practice until 2004 are generally not compatible with the directive.

Spotlight on policy: European Working Time Directive – *continued*

New working practices to ensure compliance are likely to include:

- development of emergency medical teams providing cover across a hospital at night
- new non-medical roles supporting and substituting for doctors in training
- fewer tiers of emergency medical cover
- new service models
- new teamworking patterns.

Although the directive has provided the impetus for change, it is more than a human resources issue. Complying with it must be seen as part of a wider opportunity to redesign service delivery and improve work-life balance for NHS staff. Implementing the directive will affect the design and delivery of all acute health services, and gives the NHS the chance to provide services in ways that are more responsive to the needs of patients and staff.

But meeting the directive's requirements, particularly the SiMAP and Jaeger judgements, will be a real challenge for the NHS. Some organisations may not be able to continue to provide current services and comply.

Further information

Briefing 101: The European Working Time Directive, NHS Confederation, May 2004.

Workforce planning

Workforce planning in the NHS has undergone major reorganisation, stemming from long-standing concerns about the way in which the NHS educated, trained and used its staff. It was generally felt that workforce planning was not built around service needs and the skills required to deliver them, nor was it well integrated with service and financial planning. It failed to look across primary, secondary and tertiary care or across staff groups, and was insufficiently responsive to changes and developments. There was little multidisciplinary training, education and working.

Reforms have aimed at securing greater integration, more flexibility, better management ownership, clearer roles and responsibilities, improved training, education and regulation, increased staff numbers and clear and flexible career structures and pathways.

Key text: ***A health service of all the talents: developing the NHS workforce***

This is a consultation document on the review of workforce planning, published in April 2000. Its theme is 'that the NHS workforce, whose commitment no one can doubt, needs to be transformed in order to provide the sort of care which will be needed in the future'. It emphasised:

- teamworking across professional and organisational boundaries
- flexible working to make the best use of the range of staff skills and knowledge
- streamlined workforce planning and development based on patients' needs, not professionals'
- maximising the contribution of all staff to patient care, doing away with barriers which say only doctors or nurses can provide particular types of care
- modernising education and training to ensure staff are equipped with the skills to work in a complex, changing NHS
- developing new, more flexible, careers for staff of all professions
- expanding the workforce to meet future demands.

Workforce development confederations

Workforce development confederations (WDCs) were set up in 2001 to bring together local NHS and non-NHS employers to plan and develop the whole healthcare workforce. This reflects the fact that the NHS is not the only employer of healthcare staff, and that local authorities, private and voluntary sector providers and others need to work together if workforce planning and development is to be effective. They have since been integrated with strategic health authorities.

The local membership of WDCs comprises representatives from:

- NHS trusts
- primary care trusts
- ambulance trusts
- care trusts
- postgraduate deaneries
- councils with social services departments and other social care employers
- further and higher education institutions
- independent sector organisations
- learning and skills councils
- Ministry of Defence
- National Blood Authority

- NHS Direct
- Prison Service
- voluntary sector organisations.

They need to work closely with Government Offices for the Regions (see page 134) and regional development agencies to ensure their plans reflect wider labour market issues.

WDCs are responsible for:
- developing the existing and future workforce
- developing and leading an integrated approach to workforce planning for health and social care communities
- leading in developing a shared approach to HR policy and practice
- establishing robust working relationships with NHSU
- negotiating, managing and monitoring contracts with education and training providers, and supporting the modernisation of professional preparation, education and training
- practice placements for all students on NHS and HEFCE-funded healthcare training programmes
- promoting patient, carer and student input into healthcare education and training
- co-ordinating the strategic management of local learning and education facilities and their revenue consequences.

Further information
www.wdc.nhs.uk

Changing Workforce Programme
The Changing Workforce Programme run by the NHS Modernisation Agency's New Ways of Working Team, is helping the NHS and other health and social care organisations to redesign staff roles. It is working locally and nationally to enable role redesign to become mainstream, spreading lessons from 17 pilot sites that have tested and implemented role redesign.

The programme's role redesign workshop provides skills and tools to implement new or redesigned roles. The role redesign database and advice line (0845 600 0700) are aimed at anyone wishing to learn how to develop and implement role redesign.

Electronic staff record project

The electronic staff record (ESR) project will replace 29 payroll and 38 HR systems with a single, national, integrated system to be used by all 650 NHS organisations in England and Wales. It will store 1.2 million NHS employee records, covering 7 per cent of the UK working population. Up to 20,400 users will be able to access the system at the same time.

Employee data will need to be entered only once and will move when the employee moves, avoiding multiple data entry. The benefits of ESR should include less duplication of effort, greater time savings and more reliable data.

The system will be able to handle:

- recruitment
- training administration
- bank administration
- absence
- career management.

Optional modules will handle time, attendance and rostering, occupational health and risk management, employee self-service and line-manager access.

The ESR will assist workforce planning nationally and regionally, and enable better comparisons of HR and payroll data. But the full range of benefits will only be possible if current work processes undergo significant change.

By the end of 2004, 15 pilot organisations are expected to have implemented ESR.

Further information

www.esrsolution.co.uk/index.htm

8 Information technology in the NHS

The NHS will invest £2.3 billion in information technology over the next three years in an ambitious programme to revolutionise its IT capability. Currently, most NHS trusts have multiple, separate IT systems, each with their own patient data/record base. Even within the same trust, separate systems often support separate patient records that do not communicate with each other. Similarly in primary care, individual practices have their own applications, so patient records cannot be easily transferred.

Modern information systems will enable the NHS to change fundamentally the way care is delivered, improve quality and use resources more effectively. Many in the service have long recognised this as essential, but it has proved difficult to achieve. All the proposed changes are technically feasible individually, but have never been integrated anywhere in the world. It is seen as the 'IT challenge of the decade'.

The Wanless Report in 2002 made several key recommendations for IT in the NHS:

- doubling the IT budget and ensuring that funding is not used to subsidise other services
- stringent, centrally managed national standards for data and IT
- better management of IT implementation, including a national programme.

Wanless underlined the fact that the NHS Plan's targets and modernisation objectives require a new approach to information and communications technology: 'Without a major advance in the effective use of ICT, the health service will find it increasingly difficult to deliver the efficient, high-quality service which the public will demand. This is a major priority which will have a crucial impact on the health service over future years.'

The Wanless Report coincided with *Delivering the NHS Plan,* which proposed offering patients more choice. The new IT strategy outlined in *Delivering 21st-century IT support for the NHS – a national strategic programme* synthesised elements of both.

National Programme for IT

The National Programme for IT in the NHS focuses on four key developments that will make a significant difference to services:

- an underpinning IT infrastructure with sufficient connectivity and broadband capacity to support the critical national applications and local systems.
- electronic appointment booking
- an electronic care records service
- electronic transmission of prescriptions.

The programme, based in the Department of Health in London and Leeds, comprises a team of about 150 procurement and project management experts who are leading implementation of the IT strategy. The programme is headed by the director general of NHS IT and is directed by a national programme board that includes representatives from across Government. It has:

- a ministerial taskforce overseeing its strategic direction
- a director general to lead and ensure delivery of the national components and co-ordinate local implementation
- nationally held resources
- stringent national standards for data and IT in the NHS
- a national procurement strategy to accelerate the impact of IT across the service
- an improved partnership with the industry nationally, involving a small number of local service providers.

Further information

Briefing 88: The national strategy for IT in the NHS, NHS Confederation, August 2003.
Briefing 89: National programme for IT – an interview with Richard Granger and Peter Hutton, NHS Confederation, September 2003.

Electronic booking

Electronic booking will underpin the Government's policy of enabling patients to choose which hospital to attend at a date and time to suit them. New software will be available to more than 30,000 GPs connecting them to 270 acute, community or mental health hospitals, so that patients can exercise this choice when their GP refers them to hospital.

The system will be introduced throughout the NHS in England with the first electronic bookings in summer 2004. National implementation is expected to be complete by the end of 2005. Redesigning processes to make booked appointments possible has been under way since 1998, and every acute trust now offers them in at least two high-volume specialities or procedures.

Electronic booking is likely to reduce the number of patients unable to attend their appointments, as those who have a choice are more likely to keep it. This in turn will lead to more efficient use of NHS time, as patients will no longer need to make follow-up appointments with their GPs simply to ask the progress of their referral.

Other benefits include GPs and hospital consultants being able to correspond electronically about specific cases.

Further information

Briefing 96: Electronic booking – an initial guide to implementation, NHS Confederation, March 2004.

NHS Care Records Service

A single electronic record system to which all care providers have access is essential because patients attend various institutions at different times, encountering a range of care professionals and organisations including social services and the independent sector. The NHS Care Records Service will connect more than 30,000 GPs and 270 acute, community and mental health trusts in a single, secure national system, providing all 50 million NHS patients in England with an individual electronic care record detailing key treatments in the health service or social care.

All doctors, nurses and allied health professionals with a legitimate need for access will be able to view patient information 24 hours a day, seven days a week. It will be used for:

- routine single and multiple episodes of care
- emergency and unscheduled care
- care pathways, such as national service frameworks
- telecare and services such as NHS Direct.

By late 2004, new care records will contain basic patient information and health details. In time, more information will be added, and eventually patients will be able to access their record themselves.

The design and roll-out of the NHS Care Records Service has been organised in two parts. Services that are common to all users nationally will be the responsibility of the national application service provider. Services delivered locally will be the responsibility of five local service providers, each serving a cluster of strategic health authorities.

Electronic transmission of prescriptions (ETP)

The three projects piloting ETP were set up to test different approaches to transmitting prescriptions between GPs, community pharmacies and the Prescription Pricing Authority. Each was designed and financed by the commercial sector. ETP is expected to produce significant benefits for patients, including fewer trips to the GP surgery to collect repeat prescriptions and an end to illegible and incomplete prescriptions.

Pharmacies in the three pilots included a mix of independent, small and large multiple sites, operating in urban, suburban and rural areas. Key findings are that ETP is technically viable, could provide benefits including improved patient choice and safety, and would be acceptable to patients, pharmacists and GPs.

Ministers say they are committed to ETP and are currently considering the best way to develop a secure and sustainable national service. A decision is expected soon.

Key texts

Information for health: an information strategy for the modern NHS

Published in September 1998, this is the foundation of much subsequent NHS IT strategy. It introduced the concept of lifelong electronic health records for everyone and round-the-clock online access for all NHS clinicians to patient records and information about best clinical practice. It also announced the setting up of the National electronic Library for Health.

Building the information core: implementing the NHS Plan

Published in January 2001, this preserved the principles, objectives and direction of travel set by the original strategy, but outlined how translating the NHS Plan into practice required new thinking about how to make the best use of IT. It described the infrastructure needed to deliver the Plan and support patient-centred services.

Key texts – *continued*

Delivering 21st-century IT support for the NHS – a national strategic programme

In June 2002 the DoH published this new strategy, which set up the National Programme for IT. The key change of direction was greater central control over the strategy's specification, procurement, resource management, performance management and implementation. The document reiterated that IT will now be designed and delivered around the needs of the patient, shifting from systems running along institutional lines, dealing with only a portion of patient interactions, to whole health and social care community systems that track and record an entire patient journey.

Key organisations

NHS Design Authority

This is part of the National Programme for IT and is responsible for the technical architecture of national IT systems, working out their specifications, ensuring they are compatible with each other and drawing on NHS and industry expertise.

Information Policy Unit

The DoH's Information Policy Unit is responsible for the development and implementation of the NHS information strategy. It prepares briefs for ministers and answers to parliamentary questions.

NHS Information Authority

NHSIA is a special health authority set up in 1999 to provide national products, services and standards to help the NHS make the most efficient and effective use of information. Its remit is to do 'what is best done nationally'. Among its aims are providing reliable and secure information infrastructure services, specialist support services for national initiatives and establishing health informatics as a national profession. It is based in Birmingham.

www.nhsia.nhs.uk

The electronic NHS

NHSnet

NHSnet is a secure national network developed exclusively for the NHS to pass information between organisations in safety. It is the largest virtual private network in Europe, providing a similar range of communication and information services to the internet.

NHSnet is connected to the internet via a managed gateway so that traffic may pass from it on to the internet and from there to any organisation with an internet connection. But NHSnet is protected from the internet by a firewall that prevents internet users accessing NHSnet.

NHSnet was upgraded in 2003 to provide broadband access. However, it is to be completely replaced by a new national network (N3), a process that will take until 2006. N3 will use broadband technology to link 18,000 NHS organisations compared to the 10,000 served by NHSnet. It will enable the NHS to benefit from new networking developments as they become available.

NHSmail

NHSmail is a secure e-mail and directory service that provides every staff member with an e-mail address for life and enables secure electronic clinical communications across NHSnet. It provides an online calendar for managing time, tasks, and resources within and across organisations, as well as internet access.

The directory, when complete, will include lists of all NHS organisations and sites, the departments within organisations, the people working within those departments and their contact details. As the directory progresses, this will be expanded to include details such as job title, job role, department and clinical speciality. Access will be restricted to NHS staff. Once finished, it will be the biggest directory of its kind in the world.

NHSweb

Websites can be hosted exclusively on NHSnet for NHS use, and are described as being on NHSweb as opposed to being on the worldwide web. NHSweb also hosts intranets for individual NHS organisations. Many trusts run intranets on NHSnet to provide internal administrative support across their sites. Users connected to other networks are blocked at the firewall and cannot access NHSweb sites, although they may send e-mails. Some commercial providers who also have an NHSnet connection to support remote management of systems are also blocked from accessing NHSweb sites.

National electronic Library for Health (NeLH)

Primarily aimed at healthcare professionals, NeLH offers NHS staff access to high-quality information resources, including a database of clinical guidelines, the Cochrane Library and virtual branch libraries, which are online communities creating and sharing content about specific topics, such as cancer, diabetes, mental health and learning difficulties. NeLH complements NHS Direct Online (see pages 30–31), the main portal for members of the public wanting health information. NeLH's resources are free to use, and most can be accessed by anyone, whether professionals or members of the public.
www.nelh.nhs.uk

nhs.uk

This is the official gateway to NHS organisations on the internet. It provides staff and the public with information about the NHS at a local and national level, including directories of all NHS organisations and the services they offer.
www.nhs.uk

NHS number

The NHS number is the common currency of NHS information. It is a unique identifier that provides a common link between a patient's records – both electronic and manual – across the NHS. It is the cornerstone of the move towards an electronic health record, and enables disparate information to be collated to build a comprehensive record of a person's health.

One significant drawback in achieving full use of the NHS number was that babies were not issued with it until their birth was registered. This resulted in delays up to six weeks, during which time they may undergo complex treatment spanning several organisations.

NHS Numbers For Babies (NN4B) was launched in 2002, which means that all patients, including babies, now have an NHS number from birth for life. NHS numbers will be put on any documentation related to the baby such as the antenatal record, the parent-held child health record and the hospital's discharge summary.
www.nhsia.nhs.uk/nnp
www.nhsia.nhs.uk/nn4b

NHS Strategic Tracing Service (NSTS)

NSTS is a national database of people, places and organisations. Its main function is to enable NHS organisations to trace NHS numbers and confirm the personal details of their patients, including date of birth, sex, date of death (where applicable), GP and practice addresses. This information is provided by primary care trusts and the Registrar of Births and Deaths (via the Office for National Statistics). It covers all patients in England and Wales. NSTS therefore has a comprehensive security and access policy, although it holds no clinical information. NHS staff can access NSTS online via NHSnet or by telephone.
www.nhsia.nhs.uk/nsts

NHS-Wide Clearing Service (NWCS)

NWCS provides a means of exchanging and processing high volumes of data between NHS organisations and the DoH for commissioning, performance management and strategic service planning. Access to the NWCS database is strictly controlled for individually specified purposes by approved organisations only.

The NWCS contract expires in March 2005, and a replacement project organised by the NHSIA is under way.
www.nhsia.nhs.uk/nwcs

Electronic recruitment service

The DoH launched an online recruitment service for the NHS at the end of 2003. It allows candidates to view job adverts and apply for positions using a single website. NHS organisations can compose and place advertisements directly on the website, and attach information packs. Candidates can use links with local NHS job sites for more information about vacancies, and make online applications. There are 46 NHS organisations piloting the scheme and full implementation will take until 2006.
www.nhs.uk/jobs

Primary Care Information Services (PRIMIS)

PRIMIS offers free help to primary care organisations to make best use of their clinical computer systems. Working through locally funded information facilitators, PRIMIS provides GP practices with training in information management skills and recording for data quality; analysis of data quality and a comparative analysis service focused on key clinical topics; feedback and interpretation of results and support in developing action plans to improve data quality. PRIMIS is funded by the NHS Information Authority and is based at Nottingham University's division of primary care.
www.primis.nhs.uk

9 Public sector partnerships

The concept of partnership has become a cornerstone of policy for modernising institutions across the whole field of civil and public life. It is one of the NHS's ten core principles, and new partnership arrangements – with local government, the voluntary and private sectors – are a central feature of health and social care policy. Partnership is no longer an add-on but the fundamental characteristic of public sector modernisation, and evidence is increasing that good partnership working improves services.

Two main influences affect the modern partnership agenda in health. The first reflects widespread dissatisfaction with the responsiveness of the NHS, local government and other agencies to the needs of patients and communities. It is hoped the synergy produced by partnership will accelerate improvements.

Health policy now interprets the concept of health as focusing far beyond the traditional reach of the NHS and social services to the wider social, environmental and economic factors affecting health, such as employment and urban deprivation. Partnerships hold out the prospect of tackling long-standing, interconnected problems more successfully than discrete policies in specific, functional areas.

The practical benefits of partnership working include:

- developing commissioning through co-operation rather than competitive tendering, so getting the best from all local groups instead of limiting choice and creating local tensions
- providing joint training to foster understanding of wider local issues and others' ways of working
- helping join up the health and government agenda on strategic planning, aligning local delivery plans with local authorities' community planning processes
- setting a framework for pooling budgets, providing joint services and developing joint strategic approaches to community involvement
- enabling joint data-gathering and developing common indicators and targets.

Further information

Getting closer: a guide to partnerships in new health policy, NHS Confederation, 2002.

Health partnerships: the policy context

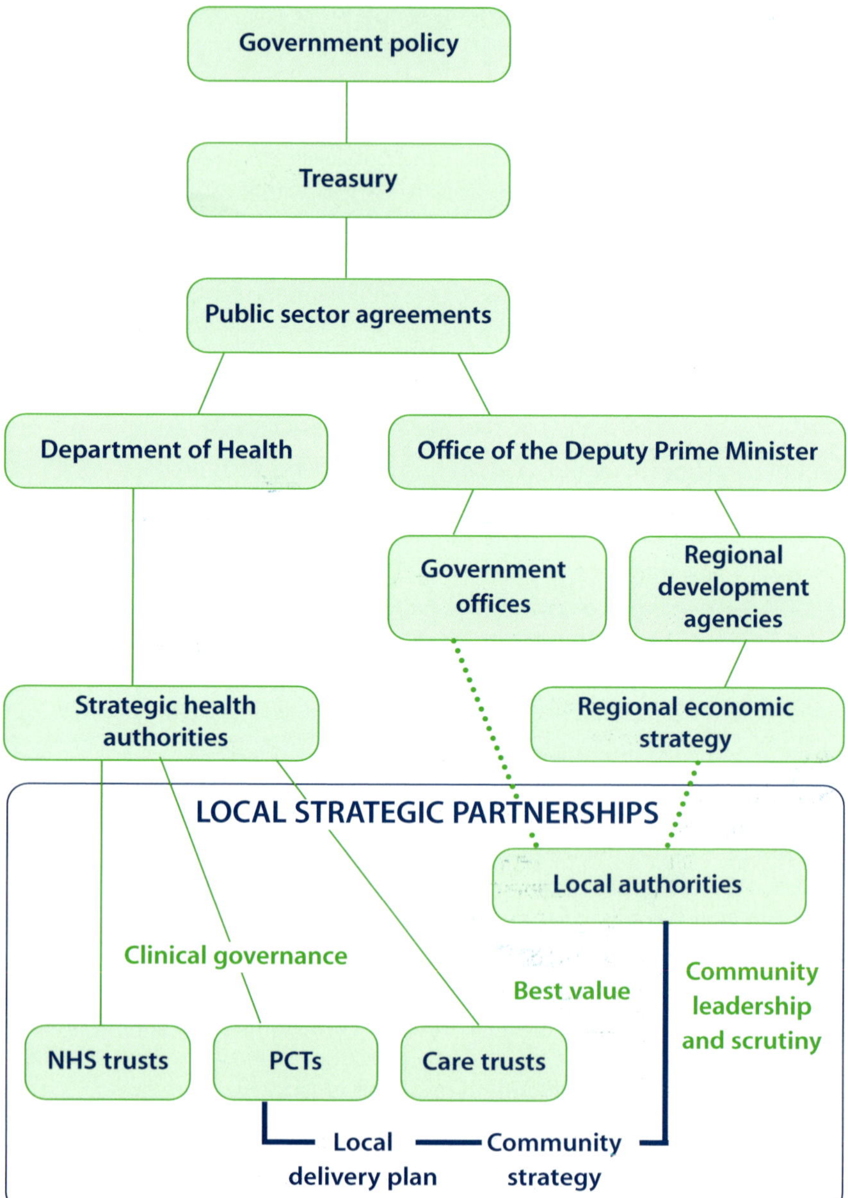

Local authorities

The Government's priorities and planning framework treats the health and social care system as one, with shared-lead priorities where both health and social care organisations have a major contribution to make. In all areas, joint working and the engagement of local authorities are required – especially in tackling health inequalities, expanding intermediate care, implementing national service frameworks, improving services for vulnerable people and neighbourhood renewal.

Encouraging co-operation through legislation

New powers to enable health and local authority partners to work together more effectively were contained in Section 31 of the 1999 Health Act and came into force in 2000.

The Act creates a new duty of co-operation between NHS bodies and local authorities in England and Wales. It provides for them to develop together local strategies for improving health and healthcare, and allows them to make joint arrangements for purchasing or providing health and health-related services – for example, social care. Strategic health authorities, primary care trusts, social services, housing, transport, leisure and library services, community and many acute services can all be involved.

Specifically, the act introduced flexibilities to enable NHS organisations and local authorities to set up:

- pooled funds – to be spent on agreed projects for designated services
- lead commissioning – they can agree to delegate commissioning of a service to one lead organisation
- integrated provision – combining staff, resources, and management structures to integrate a service from managerial level to the frontline.

PCTs have the key role in representing the NHS in developing partnerships. For this they are required to work flexibly, particularly with local authorities, which may operate on a different geography from individual PCTs. This means that in practice a network of PCTs may have to work collaboratively with an organisation or partnership.

The NHS and local government have clear, common aims, objectives and activity, much of which contributes to delivering NHS priorities. Involvement in planning, prioritising and delivering strategic planning provides ways of engaging with local communities and the voluntary sector and ensures stakeholders' involvement in NHS planning objectives.

The Children Bill, published in March 2004, enhances the NHS's role in working with local partners to safeguard children. For example, NHS trusts and local authorities can pool their children's budgets. The bill includes plans to appoint a children's commissioner for England and a statutory duty for all agencies working with children to co-operate.

Further information

www.dfes.gov.uk/childrenandfamilies

Overview and scrutiny committees (OSCs)

The Health and Social Care Act 2001 gave local authorities specific powers to scrutinise local health services and health organisations. These powers formally rest with authorities that have social services responsibilities (county, unitary, metropolitan, London borough authorities), but there are provisions for joint or delegated scrutiny.

OSCs are made up of elected council members not on the authority's executive or cabinet. They are able to call chief executives of local health organisations to attend a scrutiny hearing at least twice a year. But overview and scrutiny should be more than twice-yearly adversarial confrontations, giving an opportunity to build on existing partnership arrangements and examine services across health and local authorities. OSCs can:

- refer contested service changes to the Secretary of State
- report their recommendations locally
- insist on being consulted by the NHS over major changes to health services.

Further information

A guide to the NHS for members and officers of health scrutiny committees, DoH, November 2003.

Integrated Care Network

The Integrated Care Network is an initiative run by the DoH and NHS Modernisation Agency in partnership with the NHS Confederation, Local Government Association and others. Its purpose is to:

- lead and co-ordinate development of integrated working
- support frontline agencies working to integrate services
- increase use of the Health Act flexibilities, children's trust and care trust facilities
- support those responsible for ensuring frontline agencies deliver their objectives
- contribute to policy development
- join up working with other stakeholders, governmental and non-governmental
- maximise funding opportunities.

Further information

www.integratedcarenetwork.gov.uk

Spotlight on policy: reimbursement for delayed discharge

Over 4,000 mainly older people currently occupy acute hospital beds even though they are ready to be discharged. In about 60 per cent of cases, delays occur because social services departments have not assessed the patient for community services or because they cannot provide the services the patient needs on leaving hospital.

Better joint working between health and social care has reduced delayed discharges, but the improvement varies across the country and has been driven by top-down targeting of resources, intervention and close monitoring. The Government wants instead to put in place incentives for consistently good performance without heavy central control, so that older people are provided with seamless care, free from institutional barriers.

Under the Community Care (Delayed Discharges) Act 2003, local authorities must reimburse NHS acute trusts if social care assessments and social services are the sole reason for delaying discharge. The intention is that social services should pay for the care of an individual as soon as they become social services' responsibility, giving them an incentive to provide community services as soon as possible.

Not all patients delayed in acute beds are social services' responsibility. Some are delayed due to lack of NHS services. The type of care the patient needs when they finish their acute treatment is assessed by health and social care professionals and must be based entirely on the patient's needs.

Reimbursement places a responsibility on the NHS to start planning with social services as soon as possible. Proper assessment on admission quickly indicates whether someone is likely to need social services on leaving hospital. An incentive on the NHS to be more proactive, involving social services sooner rather than later, should improve joint working and discharge planning. Hospitals must ensure that internal processes, such as pharmacy and patient transport, can contribute to the discharge plan within this timescale.

Spotlight on policy: reimbursement for delayed discharge – *continued*

The new arrangements were introduced in January 2004. They cover acute inpatient delayed discharges only, although the Act includes discretion to extend reimbursement in future to other categories of NHS beds, such as rehabilitation, mental health and intermediate care. The Government has allocated £100 million to local authorities in England 2003–05 to help introduce reimbursement.

Further information

Consultation 8: Implementing reimbursement around discharge from hospital, NHS Confederation, August 2002.

Other partnerships

Local strategic partnerships (LSPs)

LSPs are intended to:

- bring together the different parts of the public sector and the private, business, community and voluntary sectors
- enable strategic decisions to be taken while still being close enough to individual neighbourhoods to allow decisions to be made at community level
- create strengthened, empowered, healthier and safer communities.

The NHS has a key role to play in LSPs and neighbourhood renewal by providing improving health and reducing health inequalities.

The core tasks of LSPs are to:

- develop and deliver a local neighbourhood renewal strategy to secure more jobs, better education, improved health, reduced crime and better housing, narrowing the gap between deprived neighbourhoods and the rest and contributing to the national targets to tackle deprivation
- prepare and implement a community strategy for the area, identify and deliver the most important things that need to be done, keep track of progress and keep it up to date
- bring together local plans, partnerships and initiatives to provide a forum through which mainstream service providers (local authorities, police, health services, central government agencies and bodies outside the public sector) work effectively together to meet local needs and priorities
- work with local authorities that are developing a local public service agreement to help devise and meet suitable targets.

Voluntary organisations: the Compact

The Compact is an agreement between the Government and the voluntary and community sector made in 1998. It is designed to improve their relationship for mutual advantage, with commitments on both sides. It is based on principles – such as recognising groups are independent and have the right to campaign – which have been turned into codes of practice on funding, consultation and volunteering. The national Compact ensures that voluntary and community activity is supported and encouraged, and includes black and minority ethnic groups.

Local compacts are similar agreements but at local level with councils and other public bodies. One-third of local authority areas are covered by a local compact.

Community and voluntary groups play important health roles: they support service users, act as advocates or lobbyists, provide a range of health services and are a conduit for information, particularly on health promotion. Local community groups with an interest or role in health or social care are vital sources of expertise on specialist areas.

All NHS organisations in England should now be signed up to a local compact.

Voluntary and independent sector providers of NHS and social services are now eligible for affiliate membership of the NHS Confederation.

Further information

www.thecompact.org.uk
www.nhsconfed.org/ourpriorities/affiliate_membership.asp

Government departments

A range of Government departments – apart from the DoH – have responsibilities that impinge on health, and work in partnership with the NHS. They include:

- The Office of the Deputy Prime Minister: responsible for housing, regional and local government, as well as overseeing the Social Exclusion Unit, the Neighbourhood Renewal Unit and the Government Offices for the Regions.
  www.odpm.gov.uk
- The Home Office: lead responsibility for progress on the drug strategy; the Home Secretary chairs the cross-government Cabinet ministerial sub-committee on drugs policy.
  www.homeoffice.gov.uk/tacklingdrugs
  www.drugs.gov.uk
- The Department for Education and Skills: responsible for children's social care policy and Sure Start, which aims to improve health, education and emotional

development for young children in disadvantaged areas. The Healthy Schools programme is run jointly with the DoH.
www.surestart.gov.uk
www.dfes.gov.uk

- The Department for Environment, Food and Rural Affairs: responsibilities include water, farming, fisheries and horticulture. Protection from the effects of pollution or toxic chemicals are particular concerns.
www.defra.gov.uk

Public health

Public health is concerned with improving the population's health, rather than treating the diseases of individual patients. The official definition of public health, devised by former Chief Medical Officer Sir Donald Acheson, is: 'the science and art of preventing disease, prolonging life, and promoting health through the organised efforts of society'. Many of the aims of public health can only be achieved through partnerships across Government departments and between the Government, NHS, local authorities, the private and voluntary sectors.

Public health professionals monitor the health status of the community, identify health needs, develop programmes to reduce risk and screen for early disease, control communicable disease, promote health, plan and evaluate healthcare provision and manage and implement change.

In 2004 the Government launched a major consultation on public health. In the light of the Wanless Report on public health (see below), it sought views on what changes it would be desirable for individuals, organisations, national and local government to make concerning, for example:

- restricting smoking
- encouraging walking and cycling
- access to fruit and vegetables
- food labelling
- advertising
- preventing and treating sexual infections
- healthy workplaces.

It intends to publish a public health white paper in summer 2004.

Further information

Choosing health? A consultation on action to improve people's health, DoH, March 2004.

Key text: *Securing good health for the whole population* (the Wanless report on public health)

Following Derek Wanless's 2002 report on future NHS resources (see pages 89–90), the Government asked him to look at ill-health prevention and wider determinants of health in England, and at the cost-effectiveness of action to improve the whole population's health and reduce health inequalities.

His subsequent report, published by the Treasury in 2004, argued that urgent and concerted action was needed at all levels to shift from 'a national sickness service which treats disease to a national health service which focuses on preventing it'. Random target-setting had failed to produce results, while the Government's hopes for combating obesity were unrealistic and its goals for reducing smoking unambitious, he said.

The Government should aim for California's smoking targets, and action should be taken to reduce salt in the diet, increase exercise and screen those at high risk of diabetes. The onus was on individuals to help themselves, but much more information was needed. Wanless called for a strategy led by the Government but implemented by local authorities, primary care trusts and other local organisations.

Among more than 20 recommendations were that:

- the Treasury should draw up a framework to guide ministers on what economic policies might promote better public health, such as tax credits or a tax on junk food
- the Government should draw up consistent national objectives to improve the nation's health with a three- or seven-year deadline
- PCTs, local authorities and other relevant agencies should devise local targets based on the Government's national objectives, but taking account of local needs
- the cost-effectiveness of public health strategies and treatments should be evaluated
- measures of how productive the NHS is should be based on the benefit of treatments, rather than number of operations carried out, and compare the benefits of preventing and curing ill health
- a national strategy to develop the public health workforce be devised, assessing the role of specialist practitioners and the wider health workforce.

www.hm-treasury.gov.uk/consultations_and_legislation/wanless

Public health workforce

The public health workforce comprises people in a range of disciplines who work in one of three categories:

- *health improvement and reducing inequalities:* teachers, local business leaders, managers, social workers, transport engineers, housing officers, other local government staff and the voluntary sector, as well as doctors, nurses and other healthcare professionals
- *public health practice:* health visitors, environmental health officers and community development workers, and those who use research, information, public health science or health promotion skills in specific public health fields
- *public health consultants and specialists,* who work at a strategic or senior management level or at a senior level of scientific expertise.

The public health system in England has ten core functions:

- health surveillance, monitoring and analysis
- investigation of disease outbreaks, epidemics and health risks
- establishing, designing and managing health promotion and disease prevention programmes
- enabling communities and citizens to promote health and reduce inequalities
- creating and sustaining cross-governmental and inter-sectoral partnerships to improve health and reduce inequalities
- ensuring compliance with regulations and laws to protect and promote health
- developing and maintaining a well-educated and trained, multidisciplinary public health workforce
- ensuring the effective performance of NHS services to meet goals in improving health, preventing disease and reducing inequalities
- research, development, evaluation and innovation
- quality-assuring the public health function.

Further information

Public Health electronic Library (PHeL): www.phel.gov.uk

Key organisation: Health Protection Agency

About 2,700 people work for the Health Protection Agency, with a wide variety of scientific and medical backgrounds. The HPA advises the Government on public health protection policies and programmes. It also supports the NHS and other agencies in protecting people from infectious diseases, poisons, chemical and radiological hazards. It provides a rapid response to health protection emergencies, including the deliberate release of biological, chemical, poison or radioactive substances. It works in partnership with the National Radiological Protection Board, and legislation is planned to incorporate the NRPB into the HPA.

www.hpa.org.uk

Key text: *Getting ahead of the curve: a strategy for combating infectious diseases*

This sets out an infectious diseases strategy for England and was published by the DoH in 2002. The strategy describes the scope and nature of the threat posed by infectious diseases, and establishes priorities for action to combat present as well as possible future threats. Among these measures are a local health protection service, a strengthened and expanded system of surveillance, rationalisation of microbiology laboratories, a programme of new vaccine development and plans to combat the deliberate release of biological, chemical or radiological agents.

Reducing health inequalities

This is a priority for Government because health inequalities are seen as avoidable and fundamentally unfair. Unemployment and poor housing, in particular, are major causes of ill health. Action to break the cycle of deprivation and its impact on health is central to much Government policy. Tackling health inequalities and improving health require active commitment by Government departments and groups at all levels – national, regional and local. Joint working, partnerships, networking, shared funding and resources are crucial.

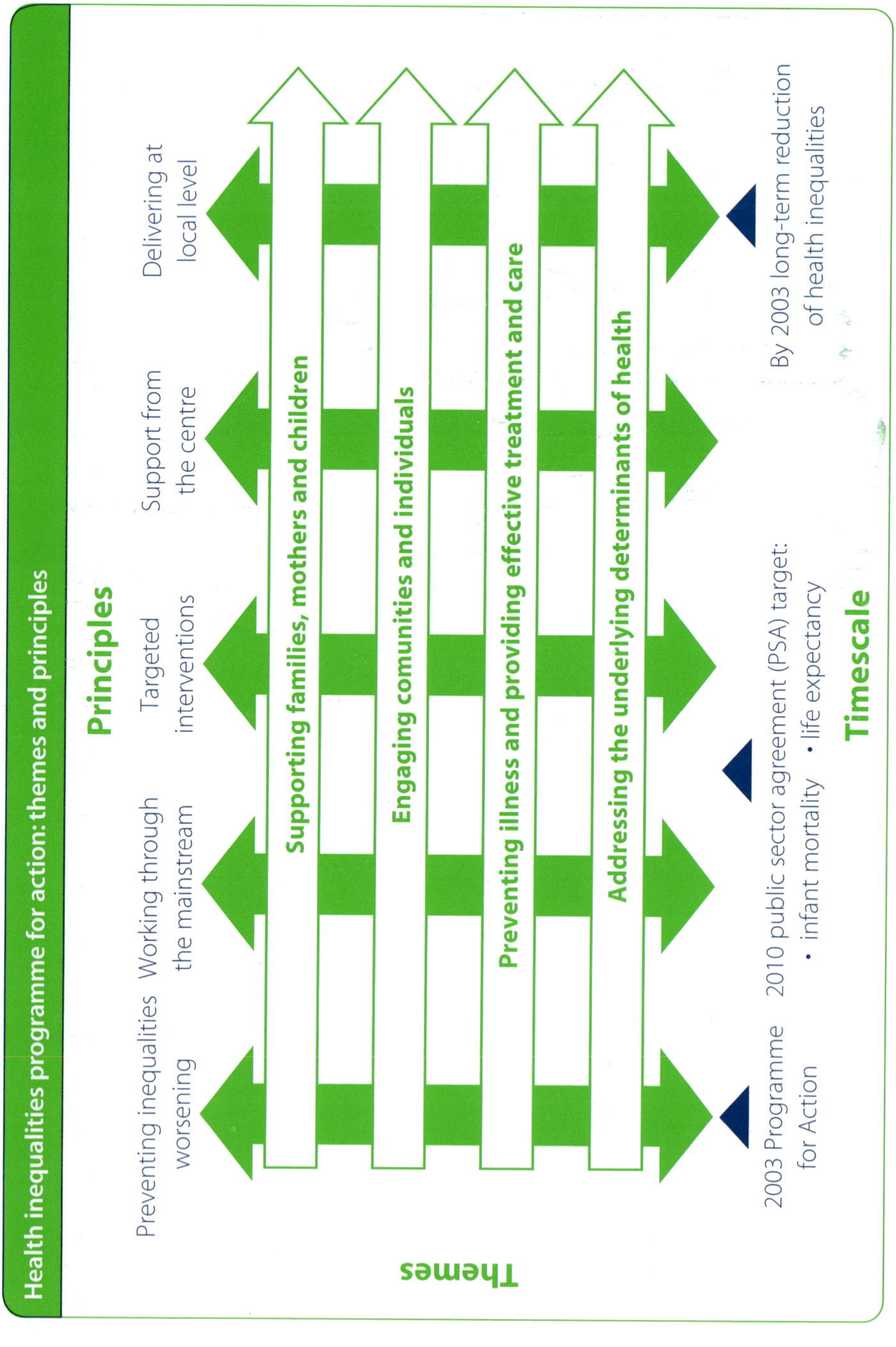
Health inequalities programme for action: themes and principles
Principles
Preventing inequalities worsening
Working through the mainstream
Targeted interventions
Support from the centre
Delivering at local level
Themes
Supporting families, mothers and children
Engaging comunities and individuals
Preventing illness and providing effective treatment and care
Addressing the underlying determinants of health
Timescale
2003 Programme for Action
2010 public sector agreement (PSA) target:
• infant mortality • life expectancy
By 2003 long-term reduction of health inequalities

The Department of Health, with the support of 11 other Government departments, published in 2003 a three-year programme of action to carry forward the recommendations in the cross-cutting review on health inequalities in the 2002 comprehensive spending review. *Tackling health inequalities – a programme for action* covers a range of local, regional and national organisations including the NHS, local authorities, social services, education, planning and employment.

Its four main themes are:

- supporting families, mothers and children to ensure the best possible start in life and break the intergenerational cycle of ill health
- engaging communities and individuals to ensure relevance, responsiveness and sustainability
- preventing illness and providing effective treatment and care by making certain the NHS provides leadership and contributes to reducing inequalities
- addressing the underlying determinants of health by dealing with the long-term causes of health inequalities.

The programme promotes the idea that organisations, staff and individuals themselves have a role to play in tackling health inequalities. It highlights three key roles for the NHS:

- leading and supporting partnerships
- ensuring that service modernisation narrows health inequalities
- contributing to the local regeneration agenda.

PCTs are responsible locally for leading partnerships and influencing partners so that their services help improve health and narrow health inequalities.

The DoH's public service agreement (see pages 49–50) contains a target to reduce inequalities in health outcomes by 10 per cent by 2010, as measured by infant mortality and life expectancy at birth. The life-expectancy element focuses on reducing the health gap between the fifth of local authority areas with the lowest life expectancy at birth and the rest of the population. The infant mortality aspect of the target seeks to reduce the gap between manual groups and the rest of the population.

Further information

Tackling health inequalities – a programme for action, DoH, July 2003.
Briefing 90: Tackling health inequalities – a programme for action, NHS Confederation, October 2003.

Key organisation: Health Development Agency

The Health Development Agency's role is to gather evidence and advise on what works to improve people's health and reduce health inequalities. It operates in partnership with a range of organisations and agencies whose remit is health improvement – not just the NHS but national and local government, the voluntary, academic and private sectors – to support informed decision making and to develop effective practice. The HDA began work in 2000, has a staff of 120 and an annual budget of £12 million.

www.hda.nhs.uk

Government Offices for the Regions

Since 2002, the DoH's regional public health teams, each with a regional public health director, have been located in the nine Government Offices for the Regions (GOs). This move was announced in the NHS Plan, which said it would 'enable regeneration of regions to embrace health as well as environment, transport and inward investment'.

The public health teams are charged with:

- developing a cross-government and cross-sector approach to tackling the wider determinants of health
- informing regional work on economic regeneration, education, employment and transport
- ensuring there is a proper health contribution to local strategic partnerships
- accountability for the protection of health (including against communicable diseases and environmental hazards) across the region
- making sure the public health function is properly managed at local level
- emergency and disaster planning and management
- being the main point of contact for serious concerns about clinical standards and associated enquiries.

The nine GOs are: North East, North West, Yorkshire and the Humber, East Midlands, West Midlands, East of England, London, South East and South West.

Further information

Nexus Management Briefing 8: Regional government, NHS Confederation, May 2003.

Public health observatories

Public health observatories are closely linked to the regional public health groups. Their job is to support local bodies by:

- monitoring health and disease trends, highlighting areas for action
- identifying gaps in health information
- advising on methods for assessing the impact of health inequalities
- drawing together information from different sources in new ways to improve health
- carrying out projects to highlight particular health issues
- evaluating progress by local agencies in improving health and reducing inequality
- looking ahead to give early warning of public health problems.

The observatories are co-ordinated by the Association for Public Health Observatories.

Further information

www.pho.org.uk

Key text: *Saving lives: our healthier nation*

This Government white paper, published in July 1999, set two major objectives: to improve the health of the population as a whole and to improve the health of the worst off in society. It announced that public health observatories would be set up in each NHS region. *Saving lives* included targets on reducing cancer, coronary heart disease and deaths from accidents and suicides, all intended to save 300,000 lives by 2010. It also dealt with wider issues such as teenage pregnancies, sexual health, food safety and water fluoridation, and announced the setting up of the Health Development Agency.

www.ohn.gov.uk

Health action zones (HAZs)

Health action zones are partnerships between the NHS, local authorities, the voluntary and private sectors and local communities. Launched by the DoH in 1998, the HAZ initiative is concerned with new ways of tackling health inequalities in some of England's most deprived areas. A central aim for HAZs is integrating their work into mainstream activity.

HAZs are part of a family of area-based initiatives: other examples include employment zones, single regeneration budgets and education action zones. However, HAZs are different from most of these in size and scope. The 26 HAZs range in population from 180,000 to 1.4 million, and cover over 13 million people in total.

The DoH has agreed funding for HAZs until 2005/06. PCTs within the HAZ areas are responsible for deciding how HAZ resources will be used and for ensuring that HAZ activities help PCTs achieve health inequality targets.

Further information

www.haznet.org.uk

Healthy Living Centres (HLCs)

The Healthy Living Centre initiative is managed by the New Opportunities Fund (see page 79) and was launched in 1999. It has a budget of £232.5 million in England from Lottery funds to develop a network of HLCs, and 350 have been funded across the UK.

The programme targets the most disadvantaged areas and groups. HLCs are expected to influence social exclusion, poor access to services and the social and economic aspects of deprivation that can contribute to health inequalities. They are expected to be accessible to 20 per cent of the population. HLCs may not be a single centre: projects can be programmes of activities based in existing premises, or services funded through mobile or outreach facilities. Local communities and users are expected to be involved in all aspects of a project.

Examples of projects include smoking cessation, dietary advice, physical activity, health screening programmes, training and skills schemes, arts programmes and complementary therapy.

Further information

New Opportunities Fund: www.nof.org.uk

10 Research and development

There are two major health research and development programmes: the Department of Health's policy research programme and the NHS R&D programme.

DoH policy research programme

The purpose of this programme is to provide a knowledge base for health, social services and other policies directed at the whole population's health. It aims to help ensure decision making is informed by all the robust scientific evidence available. The policy research programme has three priorities.

Social care for children and adults

Currently this focuses on:

- residential childcare, the Looking After Children assessment system, sexual abuse, adoption, leaving care, evaluation of the Children Act, supporting parents, costs and effectiveness of services to children in need, antisocial behaviour by young people
- evaluation of care in the community for adults: inter-agency collaboration, modelling long-term care demand for elderly people, carers, outcomes of social care, costs, and workforce issues and effectiveness of services.

Public health

Currently this focuses on:

- CJD, air pollution, hepatitis C, ultraviolet radiation, vaccines, hospital-acquired infection, fluoridation, antimicrobial resistance
- smoking, alcohol and substance misuse, sexual health, HIV/AIDS, nutrition, accidents
- inequalities in health, health promotion approaches, health impact assessment.

Strategic policy

This underpins, helps develop or evaluates national policy development relating to health services. Current programmes focus on:

- policy innovation in primary healthcare
- human resource strategies for the NHS
- information and communications technologies

- health economics and finance
- patient partnerships
- major organisational issues
- cancer and cancer screening
- mental health
- cardiovascular disease
- child health
- prescribing
- community health services for people with a range of disabilities and chronic conditions
- medical devices.

NHS R&D programme

An NHS R&D strategy has existed since 1991. Its aim is to help ensure clinical, managerial and policy decisions are based on sound information about research findings and scientific developments. Research programmes focus on the NHS's immediate needs. They are:

- **Health Technology Assessment (HTA)** – forms the largest single body of research. Health technologies include all devices, equipment, drugs and procedures across all sectors of healthcare. HTA is designed to answer the questions: does this treatment work, for whom, at what cost? How does it compare with alternative treatments?
- **Service Delivery and Organisation –** aims to produce and promote the use of research evidence about how organisation and delivery of services can be improved to increase the quality of patient care, ensure better strategic outcomes and contribute to improved health.
- **The New and Emerging Applications of Technology programme** – aims to promote and support through applied research the use of new or emerging technologies to develop healthcare products and interventions, overcoming development barriers.
- **National Primary Care Development –** aims to discover more effective evidence-based treatments and establish research as an integral element of primary care.
- **Research Methodology** – aims to promote the identification, development and use of appropriate research methods so that health and social care can be built on the best possible evidence base.
- **Consumer Involvement in R&D (INVOLVE)** – aims to improve the way that research is prioritised, commissioned, undertaken, disseminated and used.

The National Research Register records ongoing and recently completed research projects funded by, or of interest to, the NHS. Information is held on over 80,000 projects, as well as entries from the Medical Research Council's clinical trials register and details on reviews in progress collected by the NHS Centre for Reviews and Dissemination. As the most comprehensive register of current research in the NHS, it has potential to:

- identify unpublished research
- provide early warning on research which may lead to important findings
- improve uptake and participation in clinical trails
- bring together researchers in related areas
- help avoid unnecessary duplication.

Key organisations

UK Cochrane Centre

The UK Cochrane Centre (UKCC) was established in 1992 with support from NHS R&D to facilitate and co-ordinate reviews, mainly of randomised controlled trials. The UKCC currently supports over 40 collaborative review groups, which prepare, maintain and promote systematic reviews on the effects of healthcare interventions. The Cochrane Library consists of a regularly updated collection of evidence-based medicine databases, including the Cochrane database of systematic reviews, which provides high-quality information to professionals and the public.

www.cochrane.co.uk

NHS Centre for Reviews and Dissemination (CRD)

The CRD, based at York University, was set up in 1994 and provides research-based information about the effects of interventions used in health and social care. It helps to promote the use of research-based knowledge by offering rigorous and systematic reviews of research on selected topics. It also runs a dissemination service and an information and enquiry service. The CRD takes account of all relevant work, including that funded in the UK by organisations other than the NHS, and work undertaken overseas.

www.york.ac.uk/inst/crd

Key organisations – *continued*

National Knowledge Service (NKS)

NKS seeks to ensure the many sources of knowledge for patients and staff based on research, data and experience and produced or commissioned by the DoH and NHS, are brought together so that decisions can be made based on best current knowledge. It is a federation whose partners are NHS Direct Online, the National electronic Library for Health, nhs.uk, the DoH, the electronic Library for Social Care and the NHS Modernisation Agency. Its role is to ensure that information produced by its partners is of a consistent quality, and readily accessible through standard tool-sets.

www.nks.nhs.uk

Key text: *Our inheritance, our future – realising the potential of genetics in the NHS*

Genetic research will be a major factor in shaping healthcare provision over the coming generation. Genetics offers potential to improve health and healthcare through more targeted and effective use of existing drugs, as well as new gene-based drugs and therapies. Gene-based treatments will be developed in the next decade for heart disease, HIV and cancers, and could become the cornerstone of modern medicine. The Government wants the NHS to lead the world in these new developments and treatments.

This genetics white paper, published in June 2003, sets out how patients could benefit from advances in genetics, and aims to raise awareness of the potential of genetics in healthcare. It provides a plan for preparing the NHS – including investment of £50 million – to realise these benefits. New initiatives include upgrading genetics laboratories and an increase in genetics counsellors, consultants and laboratory scientists. The document also proposes a new genetics education and development centre to spearhead education and training in genetics for all healthcare staff, plus research programmes in gene therapy, pharmacogenetics and health services research.

In addition, the white paper sets out the safeguards and controls against inappropriate or unsafe use of genetics.

Further information

Briefing 91: Our inheritance, our future – the Department of Health's white paper on genetics, NHS Confederation, October 2003.

11 The NHS: a brief history

Before the NHS

At the beginning of the 20th century, a network of charitable, voluntary and local authority hospitals had developed, but it was inadequate for the needs of a rapidly growing population. The charitable and voluntary hospitals dealt mainly with serious illnesses, while municipal health services comprised maternity hospitals, hospitals for infectious diseases like smallpox and tuberculosis and hospitals for elderly, mentally ill and mentally handicapped people.

The social reformer, Beatrice Webb, is often credited with being the first to call for a national health service, in 1909. A compromise was achieved in the 1911 National Insurance Act, under which wage-earners below a certain income received sickness benefit and treatment from doctors who contracted their services to local 'panels'. Workers' families were not covered. Outside the scheme, medical treatment had to be paid for – often according to what the patient could afford. As a result, many hospitals were brought to the brink of financial ruin.

Over the next 30 years, several developments paved the way for the NHS. In 1919 the Ministry of Health was established. In the following year, the Dawson Report called for a single authority to oversee a comprehensive medical treatment system. Gradually throughout the 1920s and 1930s, the idea of a national system of publicly funded healthcare began to gain momentum.

With the outbreak of war it became a national priority, and the Emergency Medical Service was set up, giving the Government control over voluntary and municipal hospitals as well as responsibility for their funding. In 1942 the Beveridge Report described a vision for welfare reform based on eradication of the five giants of idleness, squalor, hunger, disease and ignorance. The coalition Government's 1944 white paper stated that the aims of a new health service would be:

> to ensure that in future every man and woman and child can rely on getting all the advice and treatment and care which they may need in matters of personal health; that what they get shall be the best medical and other facilities available; that their getting these shall not depend on whether they can pay for them, or any other factor irrelevant to the real need.

Early days

After the war, the Attlee Government's blueprint for the NHS described a public service more ambitious than any other western democracy's. It was to be universal – covering everyone; comprehensive – offering 'all necessary forms of healthcare'; and free at the point of use – funded from taxes. The proposal aroused widespread public enthusiasm, and for many enabled access to specialist services from which they had been excluded. The then Health Minister, Aneurin Bevan, called it 'the most civilised achievement of modern government'. The country was convinced it was creating 'the finest health service in the world'.

The NHS began on 5 July 1948. All voluntary and municipal hospitals were nationalised and overseen by 14 regional hospital boards, supported by 35 teaching hospital boards, which reported directly to the Ministry of Health. These boards supervised 400 hospital management committees, while 117 executive councils ran primary care services; local authorities were responsible for community care. Hospital doctors, nurses and other staff became state employees, although GPs remained independent and contracted their services to the NHS.

In theory, Bevan's system was intended to allow provision to meet demand. But initial funding failed to take account of the problems the service inherited, the unfair distribution of resources or the need to raise standards. No one had anticipated how demand would explode once long unmet needs could be satisfied. Soon the Government introduced dental, optical and prescription charges.

With funding capped during its formative years, the NHS had to rely on efficiency gains and increases in charges to expand services. The Conservative Government commissioned an inquiry into NHS costs, but the 1956 Guillebaud Report found little justification for charges and called for more resources to modernise hospitals and community care – to no avail. The NHS's rate of growth fell behind other health services, yet by 1958 *The Times* could declare: 'The nation has good reason to be proud of the NHS.'

Reorganisation and reform

In 1962, Health Minister Enoch Powell's Hospital Plan proposed developing district general hospitals to serve populations of 125,000 in recognition that the NHS's ageing and neglected infrastructure was inadequate for modern healthcare. In the same year, the Porritt Report suggested the NHS should break down the divisions between primary, secondary and community care, but the administrative structure was to remain intact until 1974.

The major reorganisation of that year – devised by a Conservative Government, but introduced by a Labour one – saw the formation of 14 regional health authorities and 90 area health authorities, which managed 206 district management teams. Teaching hospitals lost their separate status, while family practitioner committees were set up to oversee primary care. Community health councils were introduced to represent patients. Consensus management was the ruling philosophy.

Area health authorities were short-lived, abolished in the next reorganisation of 1982 – devised and implemented by a Conservative Government – which created 192 district health authorities in their stead. Government dissatisfaction with consensus management – perceived to have given professional groups a veto over change – led to the beginning of a cultural upheaval with the Griffiths Report of 1983, which recommended general management replace consensus from top to bottom. General managers at regional, district and unit level superseded consensus management teams, while an NHS Management Board within the Department of Health co-ordinated management nationally.

Funding crises and further reform

Repeated funding crises in the late 1980s led to Prime Minister Margaret Thatcher's year-long review of the service that culminated in *Working for patients,* the 1989 white paper which heralded the introduction of the NHS internal market in 1991. The 'purchasers' of healthcare – health authorities and some GP practices that became known as 'fundholders' – were separated from the 'providers' such as hospitals, ambulance and community services, which were formed into NHS trusts with a measure of self-government to compete with each other. The NHS Management Board became the NHS Executive, regional health authorities were reduced in number and family practitioner committees were replaced with family health services authorities. In 1996, regional health authorities were swept away altogether in favour of regional offices of the NHS Executive, run by civil servants rather than NHS staff. Unified health authorities were created from the old districts and family health services authorities.

Into the 21st century

Pledging to abolish the internal market and GP fundholding on its election in 1997, the Labour Government sought a 'third way' of running the NHS, based on partnership and performance management. It involved yet more reorganisation with 500 primary care groups (later to become 300 primary care trusts, with additional powers) subsuming fundholding, and new bodies such as the National Institute for Clinical Excellence and Commission for Health Improvement taking prominent roles. Health action zones were to encourage co-operation between health and social services, while community health services trusts were generally merged with PCGs.

The persistence of funding crises led to a large NHS spending increase in the 2000 Budget and further reform outlined in the NHS Plan later that year. The Wanless review's costing of future health needs led to another massive increase in the 2002 Budget and further waves of reform. Yet more restructuring came with the advent of 28 strategic health authorities, replacing the 100 unified health authorities. Other initiatives – such as patient choice, payment by results and foundation trusts – are still working their way through the system. The DoH's role is also undergoing fundamental change as the Government seeks to devolve as much responsibility as possible to frontline NHS organisations.

Milestones

1946	NHS Act becomes law
1948	NHS begins
	First successful internal heart surgery
	Introduction of streptomycin for TB
1951	Charges for dental and optical appliances approved
1952	First prescription charge introduced
1953	Heart–lung machine invented
1954	First kidney transplant
1956	Guillebaud reports on cost of NHS
1958	Smoking identified as cause of lung cancer
	Thalidomide causes serious birth defects
1959	Polio immunisation introduced
	Mental Health Act signals reform of long-stay institutions
1961	Contraceptive pill available on the NHS
1962	The Hospital Plan published
	Porritt recommends unification of hospitals, health authorities and general practices
1963	Gillie recommends development of the primary healthcare team
1965	The BMA's Doctors' Charter calls for improved terms and conditions for GPs
1967	Health Education Council created
	Abortion Act becomes law
1968	Britain's first successful heart transplant
	Epidural pain relief developed for childbirth
1969	Test-tube fertilisation developed
	Report on mistreatment of patients at Ely Hospital, Cardiff

1973	NHS Reorganisation Bill
	First CAT scan
1974	Regional and area health authorities, family practitioner committees and community health councils established
	Free family planning on the NHS
1975	Pay rises up to 74 per cent for hospital workers
	Hospital consultants in dispute over phasing out of pay-beds
1976	Government cuts NHS spending
	Report of the Resource Allocation Working Party published
1979	Royal Commission on the NHS publishes its report
1980	Black reports on health inequalities
1982	Area health authorities abolished and 192 district health authorities created
1983	Griffiths recommends introduction of general management
	Private contractors tender for NHS cleaning, catering and laundering services
1984	AIDS virus discovered
	First general managers appointed
	'Limited list' of drugs introduced to encourage generic prescribing
1985	Cervical screening programme begins
1986	National campaign to prevent the spread of AIDS
1987	Health Education Authority replaces Health Education Council
1988	Prime Minister launches review of NHS
	Acheson recommends every district appoint a public health director
	Crown immunity from environmental legislation removed
	Griffiths reports on community care
	Department of Health and Social Security split into two separate departments
1989	*Working for patients* white paper heralds the internal market
	Ambulance staff begin pay dispute
1990	NHS and Community Care Act paves way for internal market
	New GP contract
	Family practitioner committees replaced by family health services authorities
1991	Internal market implemented
	Patient's Charter introduced

1992	Tomlinson reports on London's hospitals
	The health of the nation public health white paper published
1993	Calman reports on hospital medical staffing
	Nurse Beverly Allitt convicted of murdering four children in her care
	Trade union Unison created from merger of NUPE, NALGO and COHSE
1994	14 regional health authorities reduced to eight
1995	All NHS hospitals, ambulance and community health services now trusts
1996	Regional health authorities replaced by NHS Executive regional offices
	Family health services authorities subsumed in unified health authorities
1997	NHS Primary Care Act
	New NHS white paper published
1998	First comprehensive spending review of public services
1999	Primary care groups start work
	Health Act imposes duty of quality of care on NHS trusts
	Saving lives: our healthier nation public health white paper published
	Royal Commission on long-term care report published
	Alder Hey Hospital found to have kept children's organs removed in post-mortems without consent
2000	*NHS Plan* published
	First primary care trusts start work
	Budget promises spending increase of 6.1 per cent above inflation for four years
	GP Harold Shipman convicted of murdering 15 patients
2001	NHS Executive abolished
	Kennedy Report on the Bristol Royal Infirmary children's heart deaths published
2002	PCTs take over from PCGs
	28 strategic health authorities replace former health authorities
	DoH regional health and social care directorates abolished
	Wanless Report on future healthcare spending needs
2003	Community health councils abolished
	New GP and consultant contracts agreed
2004	First foundation trusts established

12 An A–Z of the NHS

Action on programmes – work with the professional bodies within specialities to encourage the development and spread of good practice, initially within selected pilot sites, then throughout the speciality. They began in 1999 with Action on cataracts, since when dermatology, ear, nose and throat and orthopaedics programmes have been added. General surgery, plastic surgery, urology and neurology are following.

advocacy – where a person acts as a champion for a patient or carer. An advocate could be employed to do this or it could be one of a range of people including a pharmacist, doctor, voluntary worker or a carer.

AIDS – reducing incidence of HIV infection is a Government priority. The national strategy for sexual health and HIV (2001) requires PCTs to deliver HIV services within their area.

benchmarking – a process whereby organisations identify best performers in order to improve their own performance.

best value – system of quality improvement in local government and the NHS which sets a duty to deliver services of a clear standard, covering cost and quality, by the most effective, economic and efficient means available.

Better services for vulnerable people – requires agencies to work together to produce joint investment plans for older people, adults with mental health problems, people with learning disabilities and for welfare to work for disabled people.

blood transfusion services – the responsibility of the National Blood Authority (see entry).

British Medical Association – professional association of doctors, acting as a trade union, scientific and educational body and publisher. Some 80 per cent of Britain's doctors are members.

Building capacity and partnership in care – 2001 agreement between the statutory and independent social care sector, healthcare and housing sectors about placing older people in care homes or giving them other forms of support. Government investment of £300 million over 2001–03 aimed to reduce admissions and treatment and stabilise the home care sector with longer-term commissioning.

Caldicott guardian – all NHS organisations must appoint a Caldicott guardian to safeguard the confidentiality of patient information. They must be:

- a member of the organisation's management board
- a senior health professional
- responsible for promoting clinical governance in the organisation.

Calman-Hine Report – set out in 1995 a tiered network of care for cancer patients to ensure that care is of a uniformly high standard.

Campbell Collaboration – international organisation which seeks to provide evidence of what works in public policy and of how, why and under what conditions policies work or fail. www.campbellcollaboration.org

capital charges – internal NHS charges (depreciation and interest) made against land, buildings and fixed assets.

Care Direct project – since 2002, a DoH and local council service for people over 60, their carers and relatives. It aims to make it easier for people to get information and help concerning social care, health, housing and social security benefits when they need it. There is a free phone (0800 444 000), local help-desks in pilot areas and a website. www.caredirect.gov.uk

care programme approach – ensures that PCTs and social services departments have systematic arrangements for assessing the health and social care needs of mentally ill people, and that people referred to secondary services get appropriate care, including an individual treatment plan.

Carers (Recognition and Services) Act 1995 – gives people who provide substantial care on a regular basis the right to ask for an assessment from social services.

Caring about Carers – 1999 national strategy supporting an estimated 6 million carers. Its main features are:

- grants to allow English local authorities to help carers take a break
- credits towards a second pension
- council tax reductions for more disabled people and their carers
- more carer-friendly employment policies
- support for young carers, including those at school.

case mix – the mixture of clinical conditions and severity of condition met in patients in a particular healthcare setting.

cash limit – a limit imposed by the Government on the amount of cash a public body may spend during a given financial year.

clinical audit – a cyclical measurement and evaluation by health professionals of the clinical standards they are achieving.

clinical directorate – a unit within an NHS trust providing specific clinical services, frequently led by a consultant.

Code of practice on openness – sets out the principles underlying public access to information about the NHS. The 1995 code states that NHS organisations should make available information about:

- what services are provided
- important proposals on health policies
- important decisions on public health policies
- the way in which health services are managed
- how the NHS communicates with the public
- how people can have access to their personal records.

Commission for Social Care Inspection (CSCI) – carries out work previously undertaken by the Social Services Inspectorate, the SSI/Audit Commission joint review team and the social care functions of the National Care Standards Commission.

controls assurance – a process designed to provide evidence that NHS bodies are doing their reasonable best to manage themselves so as to meet their objectives and protect patients, staff, the public and other stakeholders against risks of all kinds, covering:

- buildings, land, plant and non-medical equipment
- catering and food hygiene
- decontamination of medical devices
- emergency planning
- environmental management
- financial management
- fire safety
- governance
- health and safety
- human resources
- infection control
- information management and technology
- management of purchasing and supply
- medical equipment and devices
- medicines management
- professional advice and services
- records management
- risk management system
- security management
- transport management
- waste management.

emergency planning – plan outlining how to deal with a serious incident, such as a major road accident, rail crash, bomb incident or chemical spill. Each level and part of the NHS has an emergency plan, which must relate to the emergency plans of other agencies, such as local authorities, police and fire services.

enforcement protocol (smoking) – developed in conjunction with local authorities to reduce under-age tobacco sales. Local authorities have to take enforcement action at least once each year.

European Medicines Evaluation Agency – authorises the use of medicinal products in the European Union and works with national medicines regulatory bodies (see also Medicines and Healthcare Products Regulatory Agency).

extended schools – schools with a wider role to provide family, social care and health services.

finished consultant episode – completion of a patient's period of care under a consultant, after which they are either discharged or transferred to another consultant.

Food Standards Agency – charged with protecting health in relation to food, with powers to act throughout the food chain to develop policies. Advises consumers, ministers and the food industry on all aspects of food safety and standards.

Freedom of Information Act 2000 – all NHS bodies must set out the type of information they publish or intend to publish, the form in which it is published and details of any charges. The act will be fully in force by January 2005.

From vision to reality – 2001 report by the public health minister and chief medical officer on progress in achieving public health targets and future prospects. It describes action on cancer, coronary heart disease, mental health and health inequalities.

Funding learning and development for the healthcare workforce – 2002 DoH paper recommending a single integrated budget designed to support learning by health professionals across the board.

General Social Care Council – promotes high standards of conduct, practice and training for social workers. The Council, which began in 2001, is establishing a code of practice and a register of social care workers.

Health and Safety Commission – responsible for administering the Health and Safety At Work Act 1974. Its role is to ensure risks from work activities are properly controlled. It reviews health and safety legislation and makes proposals for changes.

Health and Safety Executive – assists the Health and Safety Commission in its functions. It has specific statutory responsibilities, including enforcement of health and safety law. Its staff includes inspectors, policy advisers, lawyers, technologists and scientific and medical experts.

health and social care awards – annual award scheme for NHS and social services staff, which recognises outstanding achievement.

health service circular (HSC) – formal method of communication between the DoH and the rest of the NHS.

health visitor – health professional working in the community, responsible for health promotion, advice and community health development. Mothers and young children tend to be their main client groups.

healthy schools initiative – launched in 1998, aims to raise the awareness of children, teachers, governors, parents and the wider community to the opportunities that exist in schools for improving health. A website and healthy schools network support the initiative.

hospital consultants – take full responsibility for the clinical care of patients. Most head a team, or firm, of doctors in training. The team may include specialist registrars and senior house officers, as well as clinical assistants, hospital practitioners, associate specialists and staff-grade doctors. Current emphasis is on consultant-provided rather than consultant-led services, with consultants providing more of the hands-on care, and for the phasing out of single-handed posts so that cover for absence can be more satisfactorily arranged.

hotel costs – the accommodation costs of keeping a patient in hospital, excluding treatment costs.

Human Fertilisation and Embryology Authority – since 1991, licenses and monitors NHS and private fertility clinics. It is charged with ensuring research is carried out responsibly.

Human Genetics Commission – since 1999, advises on the social, ethical and legal implications of developments in genetics and their likely impact on health and healthcare. It engages the public in considering these questions.

Improvement Partnership for Hospitals (IPH) – aims to deliver radical improvements by integrating and expanding service redesign work at NHS trust level. It began with four pilot sites in 2003 and plans to include all acute trusts by the end of 2005.

individual learning account – provides training and development opportunities for non-professional NHS staff.

learning disability – people with incomplete intellectual development, sometimes accompanied by social or emotional problems. The 2001 white paper *Valuing people: a new strategy for learning disability for the 21st century* aims to help people with learning disabilities to live as independently as possible. It recognises they have greater health needs than most of the population, being more likely to experience mental illness and chronic health problems such as epilepsy.

long-term care charter – *You and your services – a charter to improve services for people needing ongoing support or care* sets out what users and carers can expect if they need support from health, housing and social services. Local authorities must complete an annual satisfaction survey.

magnetic resonance imaging (MRI) – sophisticated and expensive equipment that uses magnetic fields to create diagnosable images of the body. The NHS Plan decreed a further 50 be available in the NHS.

Managing for excellence in the NHS – 2002 paper by the NHS chief executive calling for NHS management to be strengthened by:

- implementing the code of conduct for NHS managers
- supporting managers and leaders
- through investment in development
- bringing on talent to create more skilled, experienced and diverse leadership
- developing senior management and succession planning
- reducing top-down burdens and encouraging diversity.

market forces supplement – means of topping up the pay of selected staff in areas of labour market shortages.

Medicines and Healthcare Products Regulatory Agency – formed in 2003 from the merger of the Medicines Control Agency and the Medical Devices Agency. It is responsible for regulating medicines and healthcare products. Its main objective is to protect public health by ensuring medicines, healthcare products and medical equipment are safe (see also European Medicines Evaluation Agency).

medicines management – the delivery of medicines to patients based on their needs. Aims to enable patients to get maximum benefit from medicines while reducing waste, and involves pharmacists working more closely with other health professionals.

MEDLINE – an electronic database providing abstracts of thousands of biomedical studies. www.nlm.nih.gov

Mental Health Act 1983 – under review. A mental health bill proposes a framework of new powers, including care and treatment orders applied to patients in the community.

Mental Health Act code of practice – good-practice guidance for professionals and managers implementing the Mental Health Act.

Mental Health Act Commission – special health authority responsible for protecting the interests of patients detained in England and Wales.

Mental Health Act managers – NHS trust non-executive directors who have power under the 1983 Mental Health Act to admit or discharge mentally ill patients. The review of the Mental Health Act recommends removing their ability to discharge patients.

mental health grant – administered through social services and dependent on joint strategies to provide specific services.

national beds inquiry – confirmed that the NHS needed more hospital beds in the right places to work quickly and efficiently. In 2000/01 there were 135,794 general and acute NHS hospital beds in England. The NHS Plan stipulated an increase of 7,000 by 2004, 2,100 in acute wards.

National Biological Standards Board – assures the quality and safety of biological substances used in medicine, human blood derivatives, hormones and response modifiers.

National Blood Authority – manages NHS blood services and regional centres in England and north Wales. Hospitals reimburse blood centres according to the services and products they use.

National Primary Care Research and Development Centre – a multi-disciplinary centre in Manchester set up in 1995 to improve NHS primary and community healthcare by applying knowledge relevant to the funding, organisation and delivery of health services. www.npcrdc.man.ac.uk

national strategy for sexual health and HIV – published in 2001, it aims to restructure services to meet patients' needs and prevent the spread of sexually transmitted infections and HIV. It should improve care and treatment and is being backed by increased spending and a national information campaign.

National Treatment Agency (for Substance Misuse) – launched in 2001 to provide services to drug misusers through pooled budgets from health and other agencies. It is encouraging good practice, setting standards and monitoring performance.

neighbourhood renewal – *A New Commitment to Neighbourhood Renewal* (2001) a national strategy action plan, sets out a joined-up approach to tackling the social and economic problems in the most rundown neighbourhoods – including low educational achievement, crime, unemployment and poor housing. The NHS has been asked to work through local strategic partnerships to tackle the causes of illness and reduce inequalities in deprived areas. Funding is weighted to benefit these areas and modernise GP practices.

NHS central register – central database for all NHS patients. Used to monitor changes when patients move from one GP to another, and flag populations for authorised health research purposes.

NHS Plus – NHS network that provides – for a fee – occupational health services to public and private sector employers. www.nhsplus.nhs.uk

NHS social partnership forum – involves the DoH, NHS unions and employers and deals with human resources issues. All national management, staff side and employer bodies are represented.

nicotine replacement therapy – doubles the chances of smokers quitting successfully. Available on NHS prescription from 2001.

Nolan principles – seven principles governing public life drawn up by Lord Nolan's committee in 1995: selflessness, integrity, objectivity, accountability, openness, honesty and leadership. They are used to guide the appointment of non-executive directors.

palliative care – the active total care of patients whose disease no longer responds to curative treatment. Should neither hasten nor postpone death. It pays equal attention to the physical, psychological, social and spiritual aspects of care of patients and those close to them.

paramedic – ambulance personnel qualified to provide pre-hospital procedures and care.

pathology – a consultant advisory service supported by laboratory facilities where specimens of blood, urine, tissue etc, taken from patients are analysed.

patient environment action teams (PEAT) – DoH teams which since 2000 have audited progress in implementing a nationwide clean-up campaign to improve the cleanliness and environment for NHS hospital patients.

patient pathway – the route followed by the patient into, through and out of NHS and social care services. It can involve referral from primary care to hospital, visits to hospital departments and specialities, a pathway through a clinical network, or the experience of joint NHS and social care in the community.

patients' prospectus – document to be published by every primary care trust as part of the NHS Plan outlining the views they have received from patients in the previous year and the action taken as a result.

pay-bed – a bed in an NHS hospital occupied by a patient who pays the whole cost of accommodation, medical and other services.

pay review bodies – independent panels which recommend pay awards for NHS staff such as doctors and dentists, nurses and allied health professionals. Appointments to the pay review body are the responsibility of the Prime Minister. Their recommendations are submitted to the Secretary of State for Health who can authorise the proposed pay rises.

pharmaceutical industry competitiveness taskforce – set up by the Prime Minister to see what action needed to be taken to ensure the UK remained an attractive place for the industry to locate. Reported in 2001 and referred to the need to involve the industry in the development of NHS services.

Positively Diverse – a national benchmarking programme to develop the NHS workforce across local communities. It brings together NHS organisations, local government and higher education, and is looking at how to support the capacity and skills needed to respond to and deal with diversity.

Prescription Pricing Authority – a special health authority with four main functions:

- scrutiny of pricing and payment to contractors for dispensing NHS prescriptions
- provision of prescribing and dispensing information to the NHS
- management of the NHS low-income scheme
- prevention of prescribing and dispensing fraud within the NHS.

primary care investment plan – each PCT must prepare a plan covering a three-year investment cycle. The PCIP is designed to protect spending in general medical services and primary care and to assist planning for further improvement of primary care services. It must be consistent with the local delivery plan.

Pursuing Perfection (P2) – an international programme to improve outcomes for patients across whole systems. The programme is led by the Institute for Healthcare Improvement in Boston, USA, and involves more than 13 healthcare systems around the world. The Modernisation Agency leads the programme in the NHS.

quality adjusted life year (QALY) – a measure which assesses variations in the quality of life for the patient resulting from an intervention, in relation to cost and length of life. Used for measuring the clinical and cost-effectiveness of interventions.

Royal College of Nursing – the world's largest professional union of nurses. The RCN is run by nurses, it campaigns on behalf of the profession and helps to develop nursing practice and standards of care. Through the RCN Institute it provides higher education and promotes research, quality and practice development.

Royal Commission on long-term care – body that looked into the funding of long-term care for older people (*With respect to old age*, 1999).

single regeneration budget (SRB) – funding available to areas of severe need, revamped to give greater support to community development.

smoking control network – an umbrella organisation comprising health charities, the medical profession, pharmaceutical companies and Government, which campaigns to reduce smoking-related deaths.

standardised mortality ratio – the number of deaths in a given year as a percentage of those expected.

starter homes initiative – funding to help the NHS ease staffing shortages in parts of London and the south.

strategic human resources intelligence network (SHRINE) – allows NHS organisations to share information on human resources developments, disseminate good practice and seek advice and support from colleagues.

systematic review – a review of clinical literature in a particular field that has set explicit tests for whether research is valuable enough to be included in an overview of the area.

telemedicine – the use of communications systems (such as electronic networks and VDUs) to provide remote diagnosis, advice, treatment and monitoring. Being used in both primary and hospital settings.

Transfer of Undertakings (Protection of Employment) Regulations (TUPE) – 1981 regulations designed to ensure that employees transferred from one employer to another maintain employment rights.

UK Transplant – special health authority set up to register patients waiting for an organ transplant, agree rules for allocating organs, organise their transport and ensure services comply with the Human Organ Transplant Act.

Unfinished business – 2002 report by the chief medical officer on modernising the senior house officer grade. Calls for more structured training.

UNISON – public services and essential industries trade union. It represents employees in local government, healthcare, the voluntary sector and elsewhere. The largest trade union in the NHS.

whole-system planning – strategic planning and commissioning across a range of services and organisational boundaries. Deals with the impact that changes in one part of the system, whether health and social care or housing, are likely to have on other parts.

World Health Organisation – international non-governmental body, primarily concerned with promoting co-operation in strengthening health and healthcare worldwide.

13 Acronym buster

ABPI	Association of the British Pharmaceutical Industry
AC	Audit Commission
ACDA	Advisory Committee on Distinction Awards (consultants)
ACDP	Advisory Committee on Dangerous Pathogens
ACEVO	Association of Chief Executives of Voluntary Organisations
ACGT	Advisory Committee on Generic Testing
ACRA	Advisory Committee on Resource Allocation
AHHRM	Association of Healthcare Human Resource Management
AHP	allied health profession
BAMM	British Association of Medical Managers
BMA	British Medical Association
CAMHS	child and adolescent mental health services
CAT	computerised axial tomography (scan)
CCIT	(NHS Modernisation Agency) Consultant Contract Implementation Team
CDO	chief dental officer
CEMACH	Confidential Enquiry into Maternal and Child Health
CGST	(NHS) Clinical Governance Support Team
CHAI	Commission for Healthcare Audit and Inspection (previous name for the Healthcare Commission)
CHC	community health council
CHD	coronary heart disease
CHI	Commission for Health Improvement
CHIQ	Centre for Health Information Quality
CIMP	Clinical information management programme
CIO	chief information officer
CIP	cost improvement programme

CMD	continuing medical development
CMHT	community mental health team
CMO	chief medical officer
CNO	chief nursing officer
CNST	Clinical Negligence Scheme for Trusts
COMEAP	Committee on the Medical Effects of Air Pollutants
COMPARE	Committee on Medical Aspects of Radiation in the Environment
CPA	care programme approach
CPD	continuing professional development
CPPIH	Commission for Patient and Public Involvement in Health
CRD	(NHS) Centre for Research and Dissemination
CPR	Child Protection Register
CRHP	Council for the Regulation of Healthcare Professionals
CSM	Committee on the Safety of Medicines
CSR	comprehensive spending review
CTO	compulsory treatment order
DDRB	doctors and dentists (pay) review body
DFT	distance from target
DH or DoH	Department of Health
DHSC	Directorate of Health and Social Care
DPB	Dental Practice Board
DSU	day surgery unit
DTC	diagnosis and treatment centre
EBH	evidence-based healthcare
EBM	evidence-based medicine
EBS	emergency bed service
ECR	extra-contractual referral
EFL	external financing limit
e-GIF	(electronic) Government Interoperability Framework
EHR	electronic health record
ENT	ear, nose and throat
EO	employers' organisation

EPR	electronic patient record
ERDIP	Electronic Record Development and Implementation Programme
ESR	electronic staff record
ETP	electronic transmission of prescriptions
EWTD	European working-time directive
FCE	finished consultant episode
FMP	financial management programme
GDC	General Dental Council
GMC	General Medical Council
GMS	general medical services
GPSI	general practitioner with a special interest
GSCC	General Social Care Council
GTAC	Gene Therapy Advisory Committee
GWC	General Whitley Council
HAZ	health action zone
HBG	health benefit group
HCHS	hospital and community health services
HDA	Health Development Agency
HEFCE	Higher Education Funding Council for England
HES	hospital episode statistics
HFEA	Human Fertilisation and Embryology Authority
HIA	health impact assessment
HIMP	health improvement and modernisation plan
HLC	healthy living centre
HMO	health maintenance organisation (US)
HPA	Health Protection Agency
HRG	healthcare resource group
HSC	health service circular
HSCI	health service cost index
HTA	health technology assessment
IC	information commissioner
ICAS	independent complaints advocacy service

ICD	international classification of diseases
ICP	integrated care pathway
ICRS	integrated care records service
ICT	information and communication technology
ICU	intensive care unit
ILA	individual learning account
IM&T	information management and technology
IP	inpatient
IPR	individual performance review
IPU	(Department of Health) Information Policy Unit
IRP	independent reconfiguration panel
ISB	(NHS) Information Standards Board
IWL	Improving Working Lives
JIPs	joint investment plans
LAL	local authority letter
LASSL	local authority social services letter
LDP	local delivery plan
LGA	Local Government Association
LIS	local implementation strategy
LPSA	local public service agreement
LSP	local strategic partnership
LTA	long-term agreement
MCO	managed care organisation
MFS	market forces supplement
MHAC	Mental Health Act Commission
MHRA	Medicines and Healthcare Products Regulatory Agency
MHRT	mental health review tribunal
MMR	measles, mumps, rubella
MRC	Medical Research Council
MRI	magnetic resonance imaging
N3	new national network
NAO	National Audit Office

NatPaCT	National primary and care trust (development programme)
NBA	National Blood Authority
NBAP	national booked admissions programme
NBI	national beds inquiry
NCAA	National Clinical Assessment Authority
NCASP	National Clinical Audit Support Programme
NCE	national confidential enquiry
NCEPOD	National Confidential Enquiry into Perioperative Deaths
NCSC	National Care Standards Commission
NCVO	National Council for Voluntary Organisations
NDPB	non-departmental public body
NED	non-executive director
NeLH	National electronic Library for Health
NHSIA	NHS Information Authority
NHSL	NHS Logistics
NHSLA	NHS Litigation Authority
NHS LIFT	NHS Local Improvement Finance Trust
NHST	NHS trust
NHSU	NHS University
NIC	national insurance contribution
NICE	National Institute for Clinical Excellence
NIMHE	National Institute for Mental Health in England
NMC	Nursing and Midwifery Council
NOF	National Opportunities Fund
NPAT	national patients access team
NPfIT	National Programme for IT (in the NHS)
NPG	national priorities guidance
NPSA	National Patient Safety Agency
NRCI	national reference cost index
NRPB	National Radiological Protection Board
NRT	nicotine replacement therapy
NSCAG	national specialist commissioning advisory group

NSF	national service framework
NSRC	national schedule of reference costs
NSTS	NHS Strategic Tracing Service
NTA	National Treatment Agency (for Substance Misuse)
NTO	national training organisation
NWCS	NHS-wide Clearing Service
OAT	out-of-area treatment
ODP	operating department practitioner
ODPM	Office of the Deputy Prime Minister
OHE	Office of Health Economics
ONS	Office for National Statistics
OP	outpatient
OSC	(Local authority) overview and scrutiny committee
OT	occupational therapist/therapy
OTC	over-the-counter
PAC	public accounts committee
PAF	performance assessment framework
PALS	patient advice and liaison service
PCG	primary care group
PCIP	primary care investment plan
PCT	primary care trust
PEC	professional executive committee (of PCT)
PFI	private finance initiative
PHeL	Public Health electronic Library
PMETB	postgraduate medical education and training board
PMS	personal medical services
PPA	Prescription Pricing Authority
PPF	priorities and planning framework
PPIF	patient and public involvement forum
PPO	preferred provider organisation
PPP	public–private partnership
PPRS	Pharmaceutical Price Regulation Scheme

PRB	pay review body
PSA	pubic service agreement
QA	quality assurance
QALY	quality-adjusted life year
RAWP	Resource Allocation Working Party
RCN	Royal College of Nursing
RCT	randomised controlled trial
RTA	road traffic accident
SARS	severe acute respiratory syndrome
SEU	Social Exclusion Unit
SFA	statement of fees and allowances
SHA	Strategic health authority (and special health authority)
SHO	senior house officer
SHRINE	Strategic Human Resources Information Network
SLA	service level agreement
SMAC	Standing Medical Advisory Committee
SMR	standardised mortality ratio
SNMAC	Standing Nursing and Midwifery Advisory Committee
SNOMED	systematised nomenclature of medicine
SRB	single regeneration budget
SSA	standard spending assessment
SSC	shared service centre
SSI	Social Services Inspectorate
TEL	trust executive letter
VFM	value for money
WDC	workforce development confederation
WTD	working-time directive

A more complete list of acronyms and abbreviations can be found on the NHS Confederation website at www.nhsconfed.org

Index

A

A&E wait time 52, 59, 60
Academy of Medical Royal Colleges 101
accidents 78, 135, 137
accommodation 37
accountability 24, 25, 26, 49, 50, 55, 66, 67, 134
Acheson, Sir Donald 128, 145
acute trusts 17, 59
admissions 53, 59
advisory bodies 11–12
Advisory Committee on Resource Allocation 80
alcohol 137
ambulance services 36, 94, 145
ambulance trusts 17, 36, 59, 73, 110, 146
appointments 28, 29, 52, 53, 59, 60, 95, 114–15
Association for Public Health Observatories 135
Association of the British Pharmaceutical Industry 91
Audit Commission 56

B

boards
  board committees 26
  the chair 24
  chief executive 26
  duties and responsibilities 23–4
  foundation trust boards 26–7
  non-executive directors 24–5
  PCT boards and PECs 26
boards of governors 28, 42
booking systems 10
British Medical Association 70, 147

C

cancer 17, 20, 50, 53, 57, 63, 84, 135, 138
capital allocations 83
capital spending and borrowing 83–4
Care Standards Tribunal 12
care trusts 19, 110
carers 40, 43, 148
Centre for Healthcare Architecture and Design (CHAD) 37
cervical screening 60, 145
Changing Workforce Programme 111
chemical hazards 11, 128, 131
chest pain clinics 52
chief medical officer 8, 66
chief nursing officer 43
child protection 60
childcare 97, 137
children 53, 57, 63, 102, 127–8, 138
Children Act 124, 137
children's trusts 19
chronic disease management 29, 63
clinical excellence awards 106
clinical governance 10, 26, 55
clinical guidelines 62, 63, 119

clinical negligence 64, 65, 66
clinical networks 20
clinical standards 134
Cochrane Library 139
Commission for Health Improvement (CHI) 49, 56, 73, 143
Commission for Healthcare Audit and Inspection 11, 18, 56, 98
Commission for Patient and Public Involvement in Health 43, 44, 75
community health councils 42, 145, 146
community health services 33, 146
community psychiatric nurses 39
community treatment orders 41
Compact, the 127
Compensation Recovery Unit 78
complaints 42, 56, 60, 65, 67
see also under NHS quality
consultants 28, 29, 93, 94, 98, 105, 106, 145, 146, 151
Consumer Involvement in R&D (INVOLVE) 138
continuing professional development (CPD) 68, 70
coronary heart disease 50, 53, 57, 73, 84, 135
Council for the Regulation of Healthcare Professionals 67, 68

D

delayed discharge 125, 126
Dental Practice Board 32
dental services 31, 32, 61, 77
Department for Education and Skills 127, 128
Department of Health 5–8, 48, 61, 106, 140
arm's length bodies 12
board 7, 8
director for patients and the public 43
doctors' appraisal 70
European Working Time Directive 108
National Programme for IT 114
NHS strategy 48
and Partnerships UK 86
public sector agreement (PSA) 49, 50
reform 12
relocations 12
resource allocation 79
role 6, 12
Department of Trade and Industry 24, 32
design, build, finance and operate (DBFO) 84
diagnosis and treatment centres 84
distinction awards 106
doctors'
appraisal and revalidation 70
junior doctors' hours 60
training of 98, 101
drug misuse 50, 53, 60, 127

E

ear, nose and throat surgery 29
earned autonomy 62
education 79, 110, 111
elderly people *see* older people
electronic booking 114–15
electronic care records 45
electronic Library for Social Care 140
electronic staff record project 112
employers' organisation (EO) 106, 107
European Court of Justice 22, 108
European Economic Area 22, 78
European Working Time Directive 34, 108–9

Expert Advisory Group on AIDS 11
Expert Patient 44
external financing limit (EFL) 84

F

family health services 79
Family Health Services
  Appeal Authority 12
finance 76–92
  capital
    allocating capital 83
    NHS Local Improvement
    Finance Trust 86
    Private Finance Initiative (PFI) 84–5
  NHS spending 86–92
    Budget 2002 86
    efficiency savings 87
    European comparisons 89
    NHS Purchasing and
    Supply Agency 92
    Pharmaceutical Price
    Regulation Scheme 91–2
    shared financial services 90–1
  payment by results 81–2
  resource allocation 79–80
    role of PCTs 80–1
  sources of funding 76–7
    charges 77
    overseas visitors 78
    prescriptions, dental treatment,
    sight tests 77–8
    taxation 76–7
financial compensation 64–5
foundation trusts 18–19, 26–7, 42, 48, 61, 74, 144, 146
Future Healthcare Network 2

G

General Chiropractic Council 68
General Dental Council 68
general management
  training scheme 102
General Medical Council 67, 68, 70, 71, 101
general medical services 104, 106
General Optical Council 68
General Osteopathic Council 68
general practitioners (GPs) 28
  diagnostic tests 45
  GMS contract 29, 104, 146
  numbers 93, 94
  PMS pilots 29
  practice infrastructure 79, 81
  practitioners with a
  special interest 28–9
General Social Care Council 11, 150
genetics 140
GMS (general medical services) 29, 79
government departments 127–8
Government Offices for
  the Regions 111, 127, 134

H

Health Act (1999) 123, 124
health action zones 135–6
Health and Social
  Care Act (2001) 41, 124
Health Development Agency 134, 135
health impact assessment 137
health inequalities 3, 16, 50, 52, 53, 130, 131–3, 135, 137
Health Professions Council 67, 68
Health Protection Agency 11, 131
Health Service Commissioner
  (Ombudsman) 6, 74
health service cost index (HSCI) 89
Health Technology Assessment 138
health visitors 19, 33, 67, 94, 98, 151
Healthcare Commission
  (formerly CHAI) 11, 42, 56, 61, 73, 74

healthcare resource groups (HRGs) 82
HealthSpace facility 31
Healthy Living Centres (HLCs) 79, 136
Healthy Schools programme 128, 151
heart surgery 45, 51
Higgs Report (2003) 24, 25
HIV/AIDS 81, 137
hospital and community
 health services 79, 81, 87, 88
Human Fertilisation and
 Embryology Authority 11, 151
human resources 93–112
 European Working
 Time Directive 108–9
 management numbers 94–5
 pay 103–6
  new contract for consultants 105–6
  new contracts for GPs 104
  new pay structure 103–4
 role of NHS Confederation in
  employment issues 106–7
 staff numbers 93–4
 training 98–102
 workforce planning 109–12
  Changing Workforce
  Programme 111
  electronic staff record project 112
  workforce development
  confederations 110–11

I

Improving Working
 Lives standard 59, 97
Independent Complaints
 Advocacy Services (ICAS) 75
independent sector
 treatment centres (ISTCs) 21
inequalities *see* health inequalities
infectious diseases 11, 131
information management
 and technology (IM&I) 84, 104
Information Policy Unit 117
information technology 113–20
 National Programme for
 IT in the NHS 10, 114–16
  electronic booking 114–15
  electronic transmission of
  prescriptions (ETP) 116
  NHS Care Records Service 115–16
  integrated core network 124
  intermediate care 33–4, 124

J

Jaeger judgement 109

K

Kennedy Report (2001) 44, 67, 146

L

land sales 18, 62
learning disabilities 33, 80, 89,
 102, 151
local authorities 16, 17, 20, 49, 126,
 128, 135,
 see also under public sector
 partnerships
local community mental
 health team (CMHT) 38–9
local delivery plans (LDPs) 50–51, 79
local patient surveys 73
local strategic partnerships (LSPs) 126

M

market forces supplement 152
maternal health 63
maternity services 89
Medical Register 71
Medical Research Council 139
Medicines and Healthcare
 Products Regulatory Agency 11, 152

mental health 33, 38–41, 53, 57, 63, 73, 102, 126, 138
 children and adolescents 19, 60
 forensic services 39
 modernising services 40
 NHS trusts 17
 organising mental health services 38
 primary and community services 38–9
 revising mental health law 40–1
 spending on 89
Mental Health Act Commission 14, 56, 152
Mental Health Bill [draft] 40
Mental Health Review Tribunals 12
mental health teams 52
mental health trusts 59
Mental Incapacity Bill [draft] 41
midwives 45, 67, 94, 98, 102
Modernisation Board 9
mortality rates 96

N

National and Primary Care Trust Development Programme 10
National Blood Authority 14, 110, 153
National Care Standards Commission 56
National Clinical Assessment Authority 71
national clinical directors 9
National electronic Library for Health (NeLH) 116, 119, 140
National Health Service
 core principles 3–4
 history 141–6
National health service, A (White Paper, 1944) 3
National Institute for Clinical Excellence (NICE) 11, 49, 62–3, 143
National Institute for Mental Health in England 10
National Knowledge Service 140
National Local Improvement Finance Trust (LIFT) 2, 86
National Patient Safety Agency 65
national patient surveys 42, 72–3
National Primary Care Development 10, 138
National Programme for IT in the NHS *see under* information technology
National Radiological Protection Board 11, 131
National Research Register 139
National Service Framework for mental health (1999) 40
national service frameworks (NSFs) 57
national standards 6
Neighbourhood Renewal Unit 127
New and Emerging Applications of Technology programme 138
New NHS: modern, dependable, The (white paper, 1997) 54, 72
New Opportunities Fund 79, 136
new providers
 concordat with the private sector 20–1
 independent sector treatment centres (ISTCs) 21
 overseas clinical teams 22
 overseas treatment for NHS patients 22
New Ways of Working Team 10, 111
NHS Appointments Commission 25, 27
NHS Bank 87
NHS Care Records Service 115–16
NHS Centre for Reviews and Dissemination 139

NHS Confederation 25, 29,106–7, 124, 127
NHS Counter Fraud and Security Management Service 92
NHS Design Authority 117
NHS Direct 16, 30, 49, 111, 115
NHS Direct Digital TV 31
NHS Direct Online 30–1, 119, 140
NHS Estates 11, 37
NHS Executive 143, 146
NHS Executive Search 106
NHS Franchising Register of Expertise 62
NHS Information Authority 82, 117, 120
NHS Leadership Centre 9, 27, 102
NHS Litigation Authority 64, 65
NHS managers' code of conduct 72
NHS Modernisation Agency 9, 10, 60, 61, 102, 111, 124, 140
NHS number 119
NHS Numbers for Babies (NN4B) 119
NHS Patient Survey Programme Advice Centre 73
NHS Pensions Agency 11
NHS Plan 3–4, 28, 52, 93, 98
NHS Professionals 96
NHS Purchasing and Supply Agency 11, 92
NHS quality 54–75
- clinical governance 55
- collaboratives 57
- complaints
  - Independent Complaints Advocacy Services 75
  - reforming the system 73–4
- feedback from patients
  - local patient surveys 73
  - national patient surveys 72–3
- healthcare professions' responsibility for quality 66–72
  - code of conduct for NHS managers 72
  - continuing professional development 68–70
  - doctors' appraisals and revalidation 70–1
  - modernising professional self-regulation 66–7
- national service frameworks (NSFs) 57
- organisations' responsibility for quality 54
- performancer assessment framework 57–8
- star ratings 59–61

NHS Redress Scheme 64, 66
NHS Strategic Tracing Service (NSTS) 120
NHS strategy
- earned autonomy and franchising 62
- the future 61
- joining up the jigsaw of health policy 47–8
- planning framework
  - local delivery plans 50–1
  - priorities and planning framework 50
  - public service agreement 49–50
- priorities 2003–06 53
- reforming clinical negligence procedures 64–5

NHS structure
- care trusts 19
- children's trusts 19
- Department of Health 6–12
- foundation trusts 18–19
- managed clinical networks 20
- new providers 20–22
- NHS trusts 17–18

Parliament 5–6
primary care trusts 16–17
the role of boards 23–7
strategic health authories 14
NHS trusts 17–18, 19, 25, 80, 83, 87, 102, 110, 113
NHSU 99, 100, 111
NHS-wide Clearing Service (NWCS) 120
NHSmail 118
NHSnet 118
nhs.uk 119, 140
NHSweb 118
non-executive directors 23, 24–5, 26, 54
nurses 28, 29, 30, 45, 52, 67, 80
district 33
education 102
numbers 93, 94
nurse-led facilities 34
Nursing and Midwifery Council 67, 68
nutrition 137
Nutrition Forum 11

O

older people 50, 53, 57, 89, 137
Ombudsman *see* Health Service Commissioner
ophthalmology 21, 22, 28
opticians
dispensing opticians 32
ophthalmic medical practitioners 33
optometrists 32
orthopaedics 21, 22, 28, 36
Our inheritance, our future (white paper, 2003) 140
out-of-hours services 30, 79, 104
overseas clinical teams 22
overseas treatment for NHS patients 22
overview and scrutiny committees (OSCs) 42, 124

P

Parliamentary and Health Service Commissioner *see* Health Service Commissioner
Partnership Development Group 10–11
Partnerships for Health 86
Partnerships UK 86
patient advice and liaison service (PALS) 42, 43
patient and public involvement forums (PPIFs) 43, 44
patient choice 45–6, 144
Patient Environment Action Team (PEAT) 37, 154
patient focus 43, 61
pay and conditions, senior staff 25
pay structure 103–4
payment by results 81–2
PCTs *see* primary care trusts
PECs *see* professional executive committees
performance assessment 14, 52, 54 57, 58
performance ratings 73
personal medical services (PMS) contracts 29
Pharmaceutical Price Regulation Scheme 91–2
pharmacies/pharmacists 32, 77, 116
pharmacy contract 32
podiatrists 33
poisons 11, 131
policy research programme 137
Postgraduate Medical Education and Training Board (PMETB) 101
pregnancy, teenage 19, 61, 135

Prescription Pricing Authority 14, 116, 155
prescriptions 45, 77, 91, 114, 116
primary care 28-33
  community health services 33
  community pharmacies 32
  dental services 31–2
  general practitioners 28
  GMS contract 29
  NHS Direct 30
  NHS Direct Digital TV 31
  NHS Direct Online 30–1
  ophthalmic medical practitioners 33
  opticians 32–3
  PMS pilots 29
  practitioners with a special interest 28–9
  walk-in centres 30
primary care groups 49
Primary Care Information Services (PRIMIS) 120
primary care investment plan 155
primary care liaison teams 38
primary care trusts 49, 50, 54, 110
  boards 26
  commissioning 16–17
  dental services 31–2
  financial allocation 83
  performance 14
  role 16, 80–1, 123
  service agreements 17
  teaching 17
private finance initiative (PFI) 84–5, 86
private sector 20, 21, 128, 134, 135
  concordat with 20–1, 52
professional executive committees (PECs) 26
professional self-regulation 66–7
psychologists 39
public health 6, 57, 61, 137
  see also under public sector partnerships
public health observatories 135
public sector agreement (PSA) 49, 79
public sector partnerships 121–36
  local authorities 123–4
    encouraging co-operation through legislation 123–4
    Integrated Care Network 124
    overview and scrutiny committees (OSCs) 124
  other partnerships
    the Compact 127
    government departments 127–8
    local strategic partnerships 126
  the policy context 122
  public health 128–36
    Government Offices for the Regions 134
    health action zones 135–6
    public health observatories 135
    public health workforce 130
    reducing health inequalities 131–3
    Wanless Report 128, 129
  reimbursement for delayed discharge 125–6
public service agreement (PSA) 49, 133

Q
quality of care 49, 54

R
radiological hazards 11, 131
rapid-response teams 34
recruitment 34, 37, 112, 120
Registrar of Births and Deaths 120
rehabilitation 34, 126
renal services 57

research and development 79, 137–40
revalidation, doctors' 66, 71
risk management 26
Royal Colleges 9, 34, 101–2

S

SAGE 25
Saving lives: our healthier nation (white paper, 1999) 135
screening programmes 52
secondary care
  ambulance services 36
  treatment centres 35–6
Service delivery and organisation 138
Service Improvement Team 10
sexual health 32, 135, 137
shared financial services 90–1
shared service centres (SSCs) 90–1
SHRINE (strategic human resources intelligence network) 156
SiMAP ruling 108, 109
smoking 32, 52, 128, 136, 137, 149, 154, 156
social exclusion 47, 127, 136
social services 6, 50, 110, 125, 137
special health authorities 14, 95
staff
  costs 93
  electronic staff record project 112
  health 97
  morale 98
  numbers 93–4
  recruitment 34, 37, 97, 120
  training 98–102
star rating system 19, 59–62, 84
strategic health authorities (SHAs) 14, 50, 51, 62, 80, 84, 144, 146
suicide 40, 63, 135
support workers 39, 94–5
supported discharge teams 34
Sure Start 127–8
'surgi-centres' 36

T

taxation 5, 52, 76–7
technology appraisals 62, 63
Technology in Health Group 10
teenage pregnancies 19, 61, 135
temporary staff 96
therapists 19, 33, 39, 93, 98
training 79, 98–102, 110, 111, 112, 121
Treasury 24, 49, 79, 83
treatment centres 35–6, 84

U

UK Transplant 14, 156

V

voluntary organisations 127
voluntary sector 16, 17, 20, 79, 111, 127, 128, 134, 135

W

waiting lists 89
waiting times 10, 29, 45, 52, 53, 89, 90
walk-in centres 16, 30
Wanless Report 50, 89–90, 113, 128, 129, 144, 146
weighted capitation formula 80–81
Whitley Councils 104
workforce development confederations (WDCs) 51, 110–11
workforce planning and development 109–11